LAWS OF SEEING

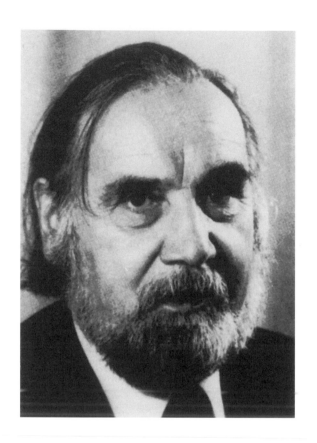

WOLFGANG METZGER
1899–1979

LAWS OF SEEING

Wolfgang Metzger

translated by Lothar Spillmann,
Steven Lehar, Mimsey Stromeyer, and
Michael Wertheimer

The MIT Press
Cambridge, Massachusetts
London, England

MIT Press books may be purchased at special quantity discounts for business or sales promotional use. For information, please email special_sales@mitpress.mit.edu or write to Special Sales Department, The MIT Press, 55 Hayward Street, Cambridge, MA 02142.

This book was set in Bembo on 3B2 by Asco Typesetters, Hong Kong. Printed and bound in the United States of America.

Library of Congress Cataloging-in-Publication Data

Metzger, Wolfgang, 1899–1979.
  [Gesetze de Sehens. English]
  Laws of seeing / Wolfgang Metzger.
    p. cm.
  ISBN 10: 0-262-13467-5 (alk. paper)
  ISBN 13: 978-0-262-13467-5
  1. Visual perception. I. Title.

BF241.M413 2006
152.14—dc22   2005058056

Gesetze des Sehens by Wolfgang Metzger published by
The Senckenberg Natural Research Society
at Frankfurt am Main
Copyright: W. Kramer & Co
1936
Verlag Waldemar Kramer GmbH, Frankfurt am Main

10 9 8 7 6 5 4 3 2 1

Contents

Much has changed in the fields of psychology and neuroscience since the original publication of Metzger's *Gesetze des Sehens* in 1936, and yet despite substantial advances in our understanding of the structural, functional, and computational properties of the brain, the study of perceptual phenomena remains the most solid basis for sensory physiology and for the understanding of why we see the way we do.

Laws of Seeing is a most remarkable book, written seventy years before our time, but covering a number of topics that are as important today as they were when it was first published. Metzger aims at overcoming the associationist psychology of English empiricism and Helmholtz's judgment theory of unconscious inferences. According to the British Empiricist philosophers (Locke, Berkeley, Hume), the brain of the neonate begins as a "tabula rasa" (blank slate), and all of the complex percepts of the adult can be traced to a history of learned associations made from the time of birth. Individual "impressions" that often occur together tend to be associated with one another, and this process of association leads to ever larger associations, culminating in the recognition of whole objects or entities in visual experience.

Although these ideas may seem dated, the key concepts behind them are still alive in today's vision research. The atomistic concept of individual sensations is captured in modern *neural network* or *connectionist* theories, whereby individual sensations are related to the activation of individual neurons, or neuron assemblies in the brain; and the laws of association between these individual elements are expressed in Hebbian learning. Yet it is hard to understand why we do not see the world as an assembly of dots (as in a pointillistic painting), but as extended areas and volumetric bodies. Only recently have neural network models begun to explain the types of continuous surfaces and solid volume percepts that Metzger describes, in a major break from earlier ideas of associationism.

Metzger circumvents this problem by confining himself to a careful description and unbiased analysis of the phenomenological properties of visual perception. Without any benefit from modern physiological methods and using simple demonstrations, he lets the observable facts speak for themselves. Based on this analysis he states that the factors governing visual perception are inherent in the visual system. Although his book contains several examples of the influence of experience on vision (notably chapter 11 on motion), the majority demonstrate that the organization of the visual field occurs essentially without our involvement. Metzger therefore calls the Gestalt laws *natural* laws. He advocates nativism, as did Ewald Hering before.

Metzger shows that it is not up to us to decide what and how we see. Rather, we already find the visual world ready-made before us. What becomes figure and ground is determined by rules according to which everything is organized without our doing. These rules are the *Gestalt factors* under the overarching principle of *Prägnanz*, which holds that stimuli organize themselves in the simplest, most symmetrical, and balanced manner. Gestalt factors are complemented by a set of tendencies ensuring that the same object in our environment changes little in perception despite large changes in illumination, distance, and viewpoint. These perceptual constancies (or invariances) are creative in the sense that they enable us to recognize objects and form experiences of the world around us regardless of the precise physical conditions under which stimuli occur.

What is most astounding is that Metzger could demonstrate the laws of seeing by careful observation of simple line drawings, paintings, animals in natural and artificial environments, and natural scenes. He points out that the same Gestalt laws that benefit human adult vision are present not only early in life, but also in the animal kingdom serving camouflage. Obviously, animals of prey and predators alike use perceptual mechanisms similar to ours. The early beginnings of ecological psychology can be found here.

The book is thus timely as many psychologists still adhere to a naive realism, believing that the world we see is the world itself. Metzger shows this to be mistaken, which is perhaps the most significant general message of the book. Three major observations supporting this message emerge from the treatise: First, there are percepts for which there is no direct correlate in the physical stimulus. Examples are brightness enhancement (simultaneous contrast) and illusory contours (bridging lines). Second, certain things are not seen although they are clearly before our eyes. Examples are objects that by their proximity and structure become part of an edge or become embedded in larger configurations (hidden objects). Third, we see objects, but differently from the way they are. This last group includes observations made under limiting stimulus conditions (microgenesis) as well as many geometric-optical illusions, where we misperceive shapes, sizes, and angles of stimuli. These observations are undeniable, they cannot be overridden by better knowledge of the actual stimulus, and they have a reality of their own.

Laws of Seeing serves many disciplines. It is written in an easy conversational style that is accessible to the academic and the layman alike. Each chapter is accompanied by a host of figures and photographs that not only illustrate the phenomena described, but also permit an immediate check based on the direct evidence of the reader's own experience. In this way the book is not just interactive, inviting readers to do research of their own as they proceed, but also highly enjoyable. After closing the book, one perceives the world with different eyes.

It makes one wonder what course research into vision and perception might have taken had this book been available to the English-speaking scientific community at the time of its writing. Many a rediscovery could have been saved, for example in the fields of shape-from-motion, depth-from-shading, context dependency, and viewpoint invariance, because the facts were known already several decades before. Take perception of isoluminant stimuli, which Susanne Liebmann[1] reported in 1929. It is astonishing to find such a treasure trove of perceptual observations that, in the English-speaking world, have been known to so few.

When discussing the *physiological route* (chapter 12), Metzger shies away from attributing the laws of seeing to the physiology of the eye, because of the inadequacy of physiological explanations and the problem of overcoming the discrete (point-like) nature of the receptor mosaic, nerve fibers, and brain cells. Many years later he would call this an *Aporie*, i.e., an unresolvable problem.[2] He also shows convincingly that eye movements cannot bring about form vision, nor can shifts of attention. At the end of his book, Metzger exclaims that "We do not bow to physiology, but rather we present challenges." Although still true, this credo has changed in modern visual psychophysics as Gestalt concepts are being increasingly integrated into mainstream neuroscience by

1. West, M., Spillmann, L., Cavanagh, P., Mollon, J. and Hamlin, S.: Susanne Liebmann in the critical zone. *Perception* 25, 1454–1495 (1996).

2. Metzger, W. (1961): Aporien der Wahrnehmung. In: Jung, R., and Kornhuber, H.-H. (eds.), *Neurophysiologie und Psychophysik des visuellen Systems* (pp. 435–443). Berlin: Springer-Verlag.

researchers proposing stimulus processing beyond the classical receptive field.

Metzger's book is a classic that will be welcomed by everyone who is interested in the past and the future of a science that attempts to relate visual stimuli to percepts by correlating them with the underlying neurophysiological processes and mechanisms. It will inspire psychophysicists to seek brain correlates of the phenomena that to this day defy explanation in terms of contemporary concepts of neural representation and computation. It will also encourage neurophysiologists to study Gestalt phenomena at the neuronal level and to think of visual perception as a holistic, global process. How often does it occur that a scientific book preserves the freshness of its early days? Metzger's *Laws of Seeing* is such a book, testifying to the renaissance of the Gestalt movement that we are witnessing in psychology and neuroscience today.

Readers may notice the paucity of references to the original Gestalt masters, Max Wertheimer, Wolfgang Köhler, Kurt Koffka, and others. Metzger clearly draws on their discoveries of the perceptual phenomena that he presents and discusses. Political considerations at the time may have precluded an explicit mentioning of the names of the first-generation theorists and their students, associated with the Berlin Gestalt school. Those missing references appear at the end of each chapter in the vastly expanded second (1954) and third (1975) editions of the book, with the third edition even dedicated to Max Wertheimer.

Some scholars have raised questions about Metzger's political past in the Third Reich and the possible appropriation of Gestalt theory by the Nazi regime. See, for example, Mitchell G. Ash's *Gestalt Psychology in German Culture 1890–1967: Holism and the Quest for Objectivity* (Cambridge: Cambridge University Press, 1995), chapter 20, pp. 346–354. This is a subject for further scholarly investigation.

The second edition contained a chapter on motion perception that was absent from the first edition, which is the one translated here. That chapter was so significant that it was translated independently by Ulric Neisser, and is available online at http://people.brandeis.edu/~sekuler/metzgerChapter/.

The translation of this remarkable book was suggested by Ken Nakayama of Harvard University. Heiko Hecht and Ellen McAfee (MIT, Universität Mainz) had already done the introduction and the first chapter when Mimsey Stromeyer (Concord, Massachusetts) took it upon herself to provide the first, inspired version of the whole book. Michael Wertheimer (University of Colorado at Boulder) followed with a revision closer to the original. Steven Lehar (Manchester, Massachusetts) changed Metzger's prose to modern style, bringing out hidden meanings where the German original was somewhat vague. The final editing was a joint effort. The book you hold in your hands is the best we could achieve short of rewriting it.

We thank MIT Press for their enthusiasm and great care in the production of the book. We also thank all our colleagues from whom we received help and moral support. John S. Werner and Walter H. Ehrenstein read the manuscript and had a pivotal role in facilitating the publication. Stephen Grossberg, Richard M. Held, Stephen E. Palmer, Peter H. Schiller, and Gerhard Stemberger took an active interest and encouraged us in many ways. We are also grateful to the anonymous reviewers for their thoughtful feedback.

The book was produced with the technical assistance of Jutta Bauer who transcribed the first, handwritten manuscript. Simon Spillmann and Kai Hamburger scanned in the figures, and Tobias Otte transferred the electronic data files. Alex Lehar helped with digital image restoration. We thank them all.

We are indebted to the University of Freiburg and the University of Colorado at Boulder for providing facilities and the German Research Council for absorbing material costs.

The financial support by the Fritz Thyssen Stiftung für Wissenschaftsförderung and the Society for Gestalt Theory and Its Applications is gratefully acknowledged.

Lothar Spillmann, Freiburg im Breisgau

PREFACE

The following chapters seek to report some of what has been achieved in our psychological institutes by experimental research in the field of perceptual science (mainly during the last twenty-five years). They seek to show that this research did not concern esoteric individual questions, but had to do with very lively matters that concern everyone. They are intended to convey an impression of the revolution in fundamental theoretical concepts, based on research in psychology, that has occurred and is still under way.

The book arose from essays that appeared individually in 1935 and 1936 in *Natur und Volk* (*Nature and People*), the journal of the Senckenberg Scientific Society in Frankfurt am Main. Some essays are completely new, and others have been revised and partly expanded in text and figures. This diverse origin, traces of which are noticeable here and there in the details as well as in the overall scheme, will certainly not weaken the book.

Without the generous cooperation of the editor of the journal, Prof. Dr. Rudolf Richter, Frankfurt am Main, some of the very difficult issues could never have been presented so clearly. My special thanks therefore go to him, as well as to my teachers, colleagues, and assistants.

Wolfgang Metzger
Frankfurt am Main, September 1936

Introduction: Overview of the History of Visual Theory

―――――

This book deals almost exclusively with external objects, their forms and colors, their substance, and their behavior. Little is said about the observer. Nevertheless it is not a physics book, but *a book about human nature*. How is this possible?

A short and greatly simplified overview of the history of visual theory may clarify this. What is dealt with are not settled issues. As readers will immediately discover for themselves, none of the early stages of development of this theory have yet been finally resolved.

1. The Everyday View

For people who naively look around, their own eyes appear to be a kind of *window*. As soon as the curtains, the eyelids, are opened there "is" a visible world of things and of other beings out there. Nothing could arouse the suspicion that any of its recognizable properties might originate *in the observer* or could be *codetermined* by the observer's nature—except perhaps for the effects of greater or lesser transparency of the "window panes." But the converse is true as well: observers do not sense an immediate external influence of seen things on their bodies unless they happen to look directly into the sun or into a smelting furnace. They can enjoy or be angry about the perceived object, feel repelled by it, or be irresistibly attracted to it, they can be surprised, lulled, or disappointed by it; but these are events that are clearly distinct from the process of seeing per se. The observer is, to be sure, not completely uninvolved in this process, as the verb "to see" in itself indicates. "To see" at this point means nothing more than being prepared, that is, open, focused, and more or less concentrated and alert. According to the everyday view, visual theory essentially deals only with eye movements and attention.

2. THE INVASION OF NATURAL SCIENCE: PERCEPTUAL THEORY AS THE THEORY OF IMPRESSIONS, THEIR RETENTION, AND THEIR CONNECTION

Sooner or later it becomes clear that not only the blinding and painful sun, but also every harmless and inconspicuous thing impinges upon the eyes, and that no vision at all is possible without these mysterious events, which even from the greatest distances manage to get from the surface of things into the eyes of the observer. Hence the structure of the eye is being studied. The theory of light, especially of refraction, is applied to it. The image of things on the rear surface of the eye, the *retinal image*, is discovered. Many characteristics of seeing now become immediately clear. In particular, some weaknesses and limitations are explicable, for example, as caused by the imperfect curvature of the light–refracting parts and the coarse granularity of the light–sensitive layer.

Moreover, it appears that above all the perceiving of a particular thing is entirely dependent on the nature of the external influence. Things such as the blank sheet of paper, on which the writer's quill leaves its traces, the wax tablet into which all kinds of signs can be impressed, and later, naturally, the photographic plate become the preferred metaphors for the seeing eye and for the perceiving human being altogether. Except for the ability to direct one's gaze, the observer's own contribution to vision seems to be confined to the fact that one is able to receive and retain impressions or other traces of the events that one encounters. Attentional relationships fit easily into this picture as intended or unintended *fluctuations in receptivity*. But these comparisons, without exception, are lame: human memory traces are not at all fixed, but can be modified. They organize and link (associate) themselves with one another, not only within one sensory modality, but also across the boundaries of different senses. However, *what* gets associated, and how firmly and permanently, again depends entirely on external conditions, above all on the simultaneous arrival of the stimuli and how often they co–occur. The human being is essentially nothing but the passive theater stage on which all this takes place.

3. THE FIRST DISCOVERY OF THE CONTRIBUTION OF HUMAN NATURE TO PERCEPTION

Colors are now recognized as the result of external influences on particular parts of the human body. They are called "sensations" in order to express that they belong together with heat or pressure, which one really feels on one's own body when touching a hot iron or carrying a heavy sack on one's back. Nevertheless it is strange that these odd sensations stubbornly seem to cling to the external surfaces of objects and cannot, not even with considerable effort, be sensed (like the pain of blinding light) as *within the eyes*. But in view of the incontrovertible evidence of physics, we cannot be fooled into thinking that light rays (and even light sources) are themselves colored. They only evoke the experience of certain colors "within" us depending on their wavelength, and therefore the colors themselves are a property of the human nature (i.e., the brain, not the external world).

For a long time this insight only served as a warning to the physicist. But it contains the germ of Kant's thought that not a single basic property of things can simply be impressed on our mind as with a stylus from the outside. The "forms of intuition" [Kant's *Anschauungsformen*], or as one could also say, the dimensions of extension in time and space, as well as the inner cohesion and continuity of individual things, their form, and their behavior; all their relationships including the relationship of cause and effect, in other words everything without exception must arise anew in us during perception, and this can occur only because the potential for it is innately present in us.

This insight never found application to specific research during Kant's time, primarily because Kant's successors (some even to this day) reversed the errors of the impressions theory into its opposite. By drawing faulty conclusions reminiscent of Baron Münchhausen's attempt to pull himself from a swamp by his own hair, they explained *the external causes of perception also as products of the human mind*, thereby *blurring* the distinction between the objective external world and its causal effects in the brain, a distinction that is indispensable for objective research.

One of the few examples of a fruitful objective elaboration is Hering's theory of color, according to which the dimensions of color experience, just like the dimensions of perceived space and time, form a stable and closed system that is also inherent in human nature. Thus— to stay within Kant's own terminology—color is also to be included among the a priori categories of intuitive forms, something Kant himself did not realize.

4. THINKING INSTEAD OF SEEING: THE THEORY OF UNCONSCIOUS INFERENCE

But the issue of the contributions of the observer to seeing remained.

Light rays have a particular amplitude and wavelength; one determines brightness, the other the hue of what one sees.[1] However, whether rays, for example, emanate from a radiating yellow source, or from a painted yellow surface by reflection is information that is not at all contained in the light rays themselves. Light rays impinge on the retina with a particular distribution, for example, in a trapezoidal form; but they also contain no information about whether they originate from a real trapezoid or from a tilted square; and they also do not convey whether it is a small square nearby or a large square far away. Nevertheless, as a rule we see all this clearly and effortlessly. This means that differences in real external objects, which certainly are lost in the light rays and in the retinal image, suddenly *reappear* in the perceived object that arises from the retinal image!

It is surprising how rigidly the proponents of the theory of impressions reacted to this blow. The fundamental principle remained unchallenged: information that is absent from the retinal image cannot appear in visual experience either. But then how do we acquire that information in experience? The answer was: we do not see that information; we only think it. We deliberate on which possible configuration is the most probable one, considering the entire circumstances and previous cases; in simple everyday cases we already know it by heart. But even in more difficult cases everything happens so silently and with such lightning speed that we neither realize what we "actually" see, nor how we judge it, but quite unconsciously take the result of our deliberations or our knowledge about the meaning of the retinal image for something that is seen. Perhaps it is akin to having read the word "tree" in a book and being so absorbed in it that, later, instead of having seen the letters T, R, E, E we believe we saw branches and leaves. Furthermore, the thought process is so irresistible that we are deprived of any possibility of ever seeing the raw image that presumably corresponds perfectly with the retinal image.

This concept was elaborated into a comprehensive perceptual theory that, besides much else, quite obviously provides an explanation, for example, of the reconstruction of spatial depth from the disparity

---

1. The eye does not respond to differences in the oscillatory plane (polarization).

between the two retinal images and their distortions with head movement. The theory of impressions is thus rescued, but at what cost? It
now suggests a cut right through the middle of a human being, a division resulting in two inherently different parts: a lower and a higher one.
The lower one belongs to nature: it contains only lifeless impression-
receiving devices whose achievements, such as seeing, are in principle
not permitted to contain anything of the person's true nature. That
which makes a humane, lively, and creative impression in seeing as
such is declared to be a superfluous extra, contributed by the powers of
the higher realm, the true, thinking soul that is thought to be external to
nature.

5. EXTRASENSORY PERCEPTION?

The next blow to the theory of impressions came, significantly, from the
boundary area between psychology and art theory.

Although the difference between a glow of light and a patch of
color cannot be conveyed by rays of light, this is even less possible for
such attributes as the cheerfulness and the kindness of a person or the
fury of a raging bull. Such attributes, if one thinks properly about the
matter, must necessarily be lost irretrievably already on the way from
the inside of the carrier of those attributes to the visible surface of its
body rather than on the way from the carrier to the observer's eye. And
yet, as a rule (not always!) these attributes are to be found in full vigor
and liveliness in seen things in quite good correspondence with reality;
in fact, especially when one is looking at living creatures, those attributes
are frequently among the essential features of what one sees there. This
holds not only for the adult, who has had the opportunity to accumu-
late experiences over many years, but also (and especially so) for the
several-week-old neonate, who, when one smiles at it, also starts to
smile. It is not helpful to say that it is an innate instinct to reply to a
smile with a smile, because, even for an instinct, the unsolved riddle remains as to how the smile of the other person ever reaches the baby if
light rays do not carry it.

It follows that, when it comes to the perception of *character traits*
and *emotional states*, the performance of our senses is almost magical.
And who will deny having ever indulged in the thought that such processes actually cannot be rationally explained; that is, that information
about emotional states must be conveyed by some special mystical, su-
pernatural, otherworldly path from one being to another, and that to

receive these messages we must possess some special as yet unknown organs besides our natural ones, perhaps some still hidden "mental eyes" or some such thing? An earlier model for such assumptions was the miracle of magnetism, whereas nowadays it is understandably the miracle of transmitting and receiving invisible electromagnetic waves.

But such assumptions have so far exclusively been defended by people who have no idea how laborious it is to pick the one right answer among a thousand imaginable and equally convincing answers to such questions. Everyone who has seriously dealt with this issue has realized that it is useless to search for hidden organs and modes of transmission before we have sufficient knowledge about the limits of the potential achievements of the known organs, in particular the eyes and ears. And this is all the more true because precisely the same effects that can emerge from a living person can also come from that person's portrait, that is, from a conglomeration of blobs of colors or grays that surely create their effect only mediated by light rays passing through the outer eye, and containing no secret transmitters of any other kind.[2] With respect to electromagnetic waves, light rays themselves are a part of that spectrum, and in our eyes we have the most exquisite receptors for them; they are distinguished from other, invisible electromagnetic rays only by their wavelength, and it is inconceivable that the selection of other wavelengths would change anything about the difficulties in conveying information that we encountered when dealing with waves of visible light.

6.   Transmission and Empathy

Science next went in the opposite direction—as we know. Based on its knowledge about the transmission of light, science simply denied that one can, among other things, also discern emotional states in objects just by looking at them. It declared that these are actually our own feelings, which we—for whatever reasons—externalize or transfer to certain parts of the visual field. Turning immediately to some less simple examples, this means that however distinctly the amorous young man senses reciprocal love, the love in reality always remains on his part; only now he is doubly in love, once (for him) with her, once (for her) with him; and the same holds in the favorable case for the girl. According

---

2. This too has been asserted, and indeed, even by a man who in his own field, architecture, represented the "new objectivity."

to this theory, if an angry bull raced up behind us, we would not only feel mortal terror (on our own account), but also destructive fury (on the bull's account); before we have transferred our own feelings of anger to the bull, we see in it nothing more than a certain *sequence of motions*, as in the little wheels of a clockwork. Just imagine the consequences if we happened to neglect to make this transfer or made a mistake in it!

For how do we manage to sense precisely the fury on the part of the bull rather than feelings of empathy, shame, or remorse—or nearer at hand, our own anxiety that, in this situation, floods us to our fingertips and hardly leaves room for anything else? Here, too many lightning-fast and unconscious reflections have been presumed: comparisons with one's own behavior in similar situations and conclusions by analogy about the appropriate emotional state.

It remained the task of an art scholar to discover a more probable way of basing the explanation on a process that, circumstances permitting, could at least be observable. If people who have no objective reason for feelings of pride sit rigidly upright, that is, assume a purely outward posture of pride, this can have the consequence that they feel something like pride inside themselves. Associated with this is that people who are really angry can, in a sort of feedback loop, pull themselves even more deeply into their anger by roaring and stomping. It is sufficient merely externally (and only suggestively) to mimic the posture of somebody else in order to feel oneself some of what the other feels. And if you see the faces of the rows of spectators during a gripping play, you will find that in many people this urge is irresistible.

But, what happens to this empathy if we ourselves have to participate; for example, if the bull is chasing us? Only a philosophy professor with spectacles as thick as a finger and a meter-long beard could still say: "Well, we only need to mimic approximately the seen 'sequence of motion' [of the raging bull] to immediately feel something like raging anger in ourselves, and we will already have what we need." To which the attentive listener will immediately add, "provided that the bull is not too close on our heels." At that point it becomes obvious: explanations of this kind can sound quite convincing only as long as one chooses the image of a musical angel as an example or, if in case of a less harmless creature, one uses a strong fence to provide the necessary peace of mind for the observer. But it is characteristic of many psychological assumptions that they are carefully protected from encounters with such dangerous examples.

7. THE GESTALT QUALITIES

It also does not at all hold that in a play we first see a meaningless pose, imitate this behavior purely externally, and only then realize (in ourselves!) that, for example, pride is behind it. It is much more the pride itself in the pose of the actor that touches us, and that is even able to infect imaginative minds. The question of how the property of pride enters our visual impression of the actor, even though it cannot be conveyed by light rays or any other means of transmission, has still not been answered. Granted that this property is not only assumed to exist, but actually does exist, and indeed exists not as something borrowed from the observer's own stock of feelings, but as an original property of the visual image itself, only one answer remains: that it has been *newly created* in the visual image.

Chr. v. Ehrenfels deserves the honor of having been the first to dare to propose this answer; thereby he became the founder of the present perceptual theory. The motivation for it came from a number of exemplary cases in which empathy theory could be applied only with difficulty and artificiality. Just as human feelings are not conveyed by waves of light or by oscillations of air, neither is the particular character or mood that we are able to perceive in nonliving structures, in buildings, mechanical devices, forms of jewelry, and, most impressive, in groups and sequences of tones. In pure cases, we are not dealing with properties of a different origin that seem to belong to these objects only because long ago, as a consequence of particular experiences, they have intruded into these structures.[3] On the contrary, these properties have *their origin in the grouping and arrangement of parts* in larger domains or *in the form or Gestalt of these domains* themselves and they belong to their innermost nature [Translators' note: they are innate, or hardwired]. Hence the name Gestalt qualities.

Character traits and emotional states that we see in other creatures are merely particularly important and impressive examples of Gestalt qualities. Now if researchers open their eyes to the fact that the perceptual field all around them, at every moment, can be populated by psychological attributes, attributes that so far they only sought and rec-

---

3. Such intrusions of foreign characteristics do of course occur; and in every individual case, it must be determined whether the property is an original or an acquired one, whereas in the past it was always immediately assumed that the latter was the case [Translators' note: i.e., these intrusions are acquired exclusively through experience].

ognized within their own self, this is by no means a return to empathy theory. Rather than the Gestalt qualities of other objects being attributed to our own feelings, the exact opposite occurs: wherever in our perception there is a Gestalt, there are Gestalt properties as well; it would be peculiar if the perceptual experience of our own self should constitute an exception to this. Following from this obvious consideration, we also want—tentatively—to view our own feelings as a special kind of Gestalt qualities. It remains to be investigated whether these are Gestalt properties of the personal self or of larger realms that contain the ego (i.e., ourselves), for example, our collective consciousness.

Yet a second misunderstanding must be removed: we cling to the idea that individual points of a seen image, except for their location, exhibit *only three properties: brightness, hue,* and *degree of saturation* of their color, corresponding to the strength, wavelength, and mixture of light rays. Yet, at the same time we admit that the *totality* of these same points may possess *properties of an entirely different kind,* for which there is no counterpart in the properties of the light rays, properties such as taut, smooth, slim, cheerful, graceful, stern, or proud. Do we not thus slide from the secure ground of science into the realm of mysticism? No, because even physicists unhesitatingly ascribe properties to atoms that they deny to their components, single electrons, protons, and neutrons, and that they also try to understand through the arrangement and interaction of these part-structures. And this is repeated in the relation of the molecule to the individual atoms of which it is composed. Never would a physicist resort to the queer thought that the molecule must sometime in the past have acquired from somewhere else those properties that cannot already be found in its individual atoms. However, to the self-same natural scientists precisely this thought seems scientifically reasonable as soon as they leave their own area and start to think about psychological questions!

8. Research Tasks of Gestalt Theory in Perceptual Theory

Even though almost a half-century has elapsed since it was introduced, the theory of the Gestalt qualities remains mired in its beginnings. It turned out that numerous preliminary questions had to be solved, above all the question of the carriers of these qualities.

Frequently, different Gestalt qualities are found in equivalent stimulus groups, and in other cases, they remain unchanged despite a changing stimulus distribution. It turns out that the issue is the properties of *seen things*, not of groups of stimuli on the retina. The question of the genesis of the seen thing from the retinal image (see section 4 above) became a burning question once again.

Meanwhile, however, a hole was torn into the impression theory by v. Ehrenfels. The hypothesis that the activity of our senses is limited to passively enduring external influences, that therefore the seen thing must correspond in all its properties with the retinal image, began to teeter. The chief motivation for the judgment theory thereby also fell away. Now it became clearer than ever how little justice had been done to the nature of seen things by an explanation according to which seen things really are almost exclusively nothing but faint thoughts. At least it was worthwhile to investigate whether external transformations, corrections, and completions of the seen things, which to date had been assumed by science to be contributions from experience or results of thought, could be explained in a less artificial way in the immediate, dynamic response of our eyes to the respective groups of stimuli. Meanwhile, Hering had made it probable that the depth of binocularly seen objects is not mentally reconstructed on the basis of the two retinal images, but, rather, that the double eye together with its attached parts of the brain is a mechanism for the immediate transformation of the two retinal images into the single spatial image we see when we open our eyes. The investigation became especially exciting, however, particularly in cases in which the supposed transformation apparently occurs *without any special mechanism*, as in seeing spatial depth monocularly. [Translators' note: Metzger lost one eye in WWI.]

But the revolution went still deeper. At first, it might seem that at least the area and boundaries of Gestalten might be determined simply by external influences: by their borders in space; by contours of the stimulated and hence activated retinal area, and in time by the beginning and end of stimulation. Under more serious scrutiny, this stance too became untenable. As long as we are awake, the visual field is characterized always and everywhere by activity; there are neither beginnings nor ends nor borders. Reference to stimulus *differences* does not solve the puzzle either. Stimulus differences that just had contour effects a moment ago do not have them any more after something has changed in a completely different part of the visual field or in the behavior of the observer. On the other hand, circumstances permitting, well-defined boundaries often pass through entirely uniformly stimulated regions. Moreover, whatever holds for boundaries and segregation of structures at rest, holds equally for the course and direction of movements and changes, and so on. External stimuli establish certain conditions for such percepts, but in every case, as we now know, they leave open infinitely many possible alternatives. Which of these is finally adopted in our vision depends once again on the active response of our senses to the stimulus, and thus depends on *laws of seeing*, that is, on laws of *human nature*.

The revolution in perceptual theory that v. Ehrenfels started with his reference to the significance of Gestalt qualities eventually touched on the simplest, most basic questions of perception that Kant (see section 3 above) dealt with: the question of the origin of all unity and coherence. But while Kant had sought only the general possibility for it within the individual, while addressing particular cases of experience in terms of the effects of external conditions, as in the impression theory, it now became probable that the laws had to be sought *inside the human* for decisions in the particular case as well.

Thus, we are finally in the research field of which the following pages are intended to provide a few small samples.

Ambiguous Figures in Our Daily Environment

Everybody is familiar with those little pictures in puzzle books with the caption: "Where is the thief?", which you twist and turn for a while until out of parts of branches, roots, leaves, and sky, all of a sudden a more or less reasonable picture of the searched for item snaps together. We only rarely have an inkling that the whole world around us is full of puzzle pictures in abundance, often more surprising than the ones the most skilled sketch artist could create. For instance, if after a long search we suddenly realize that the "misplaced" pencil has been peacefully lying in front of us the entire time.

1. The Unfamiliar Script

Who has not at one time stood in front of a gravestone or a wrought-iron gate bearing an inscription composed apparently of completely un-intelligible runelike signs? Strange hooks and spikes are linked together (figure 1), intermixed with single small rectangles, triangles, circles, and the like. Some readers will have to wrestle with an inscription composed of such runes for quite a while (figure 2), before suddenly "the scales fall from their eyes" and instead of *black* runes they see quite ordinary, only slightly thicker, *white* Roman font letters. Those who see the figure cor-rectly right away can recreate the impression of the unfamiliar rune script by rotating the book on its side so that the lines go vertically from bottom to top.

Those who first saw runes until the figure reversed itself for them can also no longer control whether they see letters or runes. It now takes quite an effort to see the rune signs again, and usually this succeeds only for the symbol that is being attended at the moment while the other signs are not runes any more, but merely spaces between the white printed letters. To recreate the initial impression, one would have to employ more powerful means, for example, as previously mentioned, to rotate the book on its side. If you have the time, you should try to read

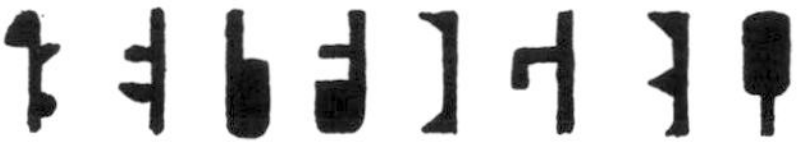

Figure 1
Individual letters of the unfamiliar script. In order to experience how this script works, begin by examining as carefully as possible the individual letters in this figure. Only afterward should you look at figure 2, and preferably before reading further in the text.

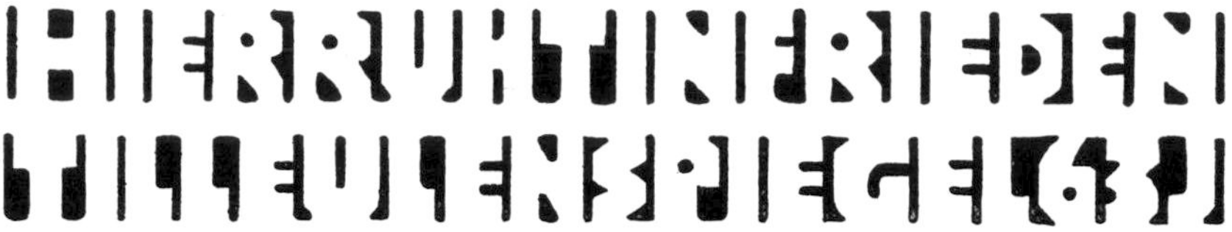

Figure 2
The puzzling inscription

often as the letters.
even though throughout our lifetime we have had them before our eyes almost as
would-be runes are intermediate spaces, the shape of which we do not recognize
is not a rune inscription at all. It consists of large Roman capital letters, and the

this inscription over and over ad nauseam. This reveals a peculiar dynamic as one interpretation becomes tired or worn out and the runes are there again in their original strength, until they suffer the same fate as the letters did before. Even if you are already quite familiar with both the runes and the Roman letters, you cannot at any moment see one or the other type of script at will, or even both at the same time. This is particularly impressive if the runes currently dominate the percept. The actual words repeatedly seem to be as if they have been extinguished, even when there is no doubt about the location at which they should appear. Such attempts, however, usually end in a general confusion in which one no longer knows what one is up to.

2.   THE MYSTERIOUS GOBLET: ARTIFICIAL AGNOSIA

The silhouette of an artfully wrought goblet (figure 3) is used for a popular classroom experiment. You suspend a large picture of this goblet in the auditorium so that students can look at it thoroughly as much as they wish during the lecture. Toward the end of the class, you ask one of the participants who has never seen the picture before to describe everything that can be seen in the picture as exactly as possible without leaving anything out. As much as you may try to pressure him that there is still

Figure 3
The mysterious goblet. The contours of the goblet have the shape of two faces facing each other. This shape is projected distinctly onto the eye—otherwise one could not see the goblet either. Nevertheless, for the naive observer it is invisible in the true sense of the term. (After Rubin: *Visuell wahrgenommene Figuren.* Copenhagen, 1921.)

something else in the picture, all he can do is to describe the goblet in greater and greater detail, and eventually declare that he has no idea of what more one might want. That there are two *faces* looking at each other does not occur to him. Those who immediately saw the two faces while reading should try the experiment with a friend.

The experience of the Roman font and the two faces offers a glimmer of what it must be like to suffer from so-called *visual agnosia*, a visual disturbance that occurs with certain occipital injuries. The eyes are healthy, visual acuity and color vision are intact, and yet somehow everything and nothing is seen. For someone with visual agnosia the page of a book is an incomprehensible swarming confusion.

3. THE FORMLESSNESS OF INTERMEDIATE SPACES

How can it be that in our examples even healthy people are temporarily agnosic, at least to certain shapes? If we see the goblet in the picture, the white to the right and left of it is air, and the air has no shape. If we see the two faces, now between them, where the goblet stood before, there is air that has no shape; and through the air you see a background that is white in the first case, black in the second; and the air is not bounded by the contour line as is the goblet (or the faces), but passes behind and actually fills out the whole rectangle of the picture, being occluded only here and there by the goblet (or the faces). Here we have the reason why at first one could not see the shape of the white parts to the right and left of the black goblet: the white is then simply a rectangle and nothing else; and conversely the black, if one sees the faces.

What we could see here with the goblet figure is not a peculiar oddity, but the manifestation of a lawfulness that governs our entire

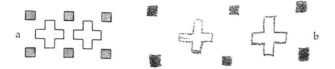

Figure 4
Cross-square pattern. If you take a brief look at the pattern (a) and draw it from memory, the figures will be reproduced fairly accurately, but the intermediate spaces will usually be incorrect (too large, b). (From H. Rupp: *Über optische Analyse. Psychol. Forschg.* 4, 1923.)

daily visual experience. Let any acquaintance who does not happen to be involved in geometry or drafting, draw figure 4a from memory after a brief inspection. If the acquaintance is not completely inept, the forms and sizes of the little crosses and squares will be fairly accurate; but in contrast, the intermediate spaces will usually be grossly inaccurate—as a rule too large, as in the drawing of a continuing-education student (figure 4b).

Try, too, to imagine what is the shape of a piece of sky that is bordered at some familiar street corner by the walls of houses with store signs and by their roofs and chimneys; or what is the shape of the piece of wall between the heads of your neighbors in an auditorium. It is clearly self-evident why seeing this shape is so difficult. But you have to appreciate that the shape of the piece of blue sky is just as distinctly projected onto the eye as the shapes of houses, signs, and trees, and *that we are nevertheless blind* to these shapes. This is just as true for almost all shapes that are projected into the eye that give the impression of an intermediate space or background. Of all shapes projected into the eye, we can usually only really *see* those that give the impression of figures, of things, of solid bodies. And, if by some coincidence, as in our examples, an object creates the impression of an intermediate space, it is as though it has been made to disappear by magic even though it is lying in plain view before our eyes. Thus on top of a messy desk, a pencil could be "hidden" even though it lies visibly in the narrow space between two books (figure 5).

4.   OBJECT AND INTERMEDIATE SPACE IN ACTING AND CRAFTING

Several known weaknesses in the way we act are closely linked to these peculiar laws of perception. Our gaze is by nature *directed toward objects*;

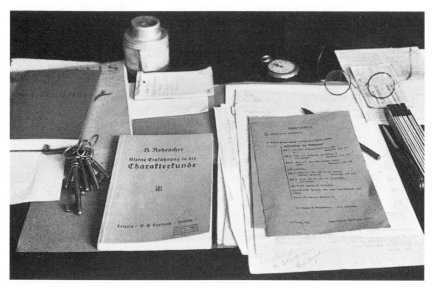

Figure 5
Mislaid pencils. One pencil is mostly occluded, the other one lies completely exposed, out in the open and does not stand out any less from the neighboring paper surfaces. But it has landed in an intermediate space and is therefore much harder to see.

one has to learn to direct it toward the intermediate spaces, the empty environment. But our body involuntarily adjusts the direction of its action in the direction of gaze (which is why an old rule says that when fencing one should look into the opponent's eyes, not at the hands). This explains the dogged steadfastness with which young bicyclists head right for a tree that they are trying to avoid, and thus cannot help staring at, even though it is the only obstacle in the entire area; and with which young soccer players hit the goalpost or the goalkeeper rather than the much larger gap in between. Certain striking features of early art can also be understood in this light. When people of the Neolithic age began to decorate their pots with line patterns, they initially worked instinctively on only those parts of the surface where patterns were supposed to appear; they were not concerned with their surroundings (figure 6a). A later stage of development in Neolithic age pottery can be easily recognized in that artists came upon the idea of letting a pattern emerge by carving the surroundings and leaving the area of pattern untouched (figure 6b). It is possible that something of this technique of leaving the background untreated was retained in certain bas-reliefs

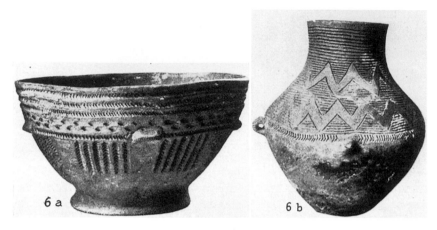

Figure 6
Two prehistoric jugs. (a) Older technique: only the pattern has been worked or tooled. (Osnabrück bowl from the Upper Megalithic or prehistoric mound-age pottery.) (b) More recent technique: the background is worked or tooled, so that the remaining unworked region becomes a figure. (Jug from Weddegast, Bernburg District, late Stone Age string pottery.) (From A. van Scheltema: *Die altnordische Kunst.* Berlin, 1924.)

often seen in Egyptian art, a style that clings particularly tenaciously to old customs. In the customary, correct technique of presenting relief (figure 7), the figures stand out from the background. To accomplish this, the material between the figures has to be scraped down to the depth of the ground. In Egyptian images (figure 8) only the figures are carved out, while their surroundings remain untouched. Thus the figures look as if they were imprinted in soft clay, even though they are really carved in stone.

5. THE ONE-SIDEDNESS OF CONTOUR LINES

That intermediate spaces as a rule have no shape, as discussed above, is related to a peculiar characteristic of seen lines: the line between two different adjacent parts of the visual field normally functions as a border for only one of its sides, but not for the other one. There are some apparent exceptions, such as the short common line segment of both hexagons in figure 9. But here one usually has the impression that at the location in question there actually is not *one*, but there are *two* boundary lines that lie on top of each other; other observers have the impression that this common boundary alternately takes turns in serving the larger

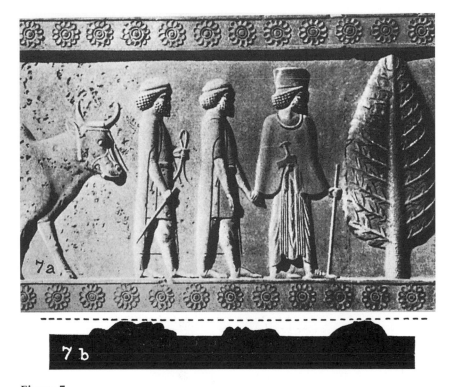

Figure 7
(a) The usual way of presenting relief in which the figures are raised above their surroundings. (Relief from the staircase to the reception hall of one of the royal palaces
in Persepolis, which were destroyed by Alexander the Great in 332 B.C.; after
"Atlantis" 1933, p. 320.) (b) Simplified cross section of a typical relief; the dotted
line represents the original thickness of the material.

and smaller hexagons. But there are in fact objects in which each single
line should serve as a boundary to both sides, as in a tiled floor or a honeycomb. Yet the unilaterality of boundaries dominates so thoroughly in
mentally handicapped people that retarded children and adults presented
with a honeycomb pattern of which they are given a beginning, as in
figure 10, cannot continue it correctly. In drawings of the most backward pupils (figures 11a and b), every line segment is so to speak already
fully occupied by serving as the boundary of one cell, so that it cannot
also take on the additional task of bounding a second neighboring cell:
all lines are drawn double. Figures 11c and d represent more advanced
achievements: here, at least for some individual parts of the boundary
lines, the double boundary role is possible after all.

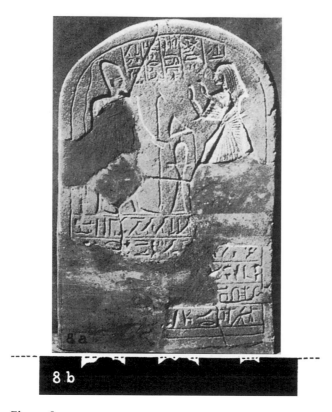

Figure 8
(a) An apparently embossed Egyptian relief; the backgrounds of the figures have
been left unworked. (Sacrificial stone of the royal scribe and treasurer Mami an Baal,
the god of gods of Sapouna, today Ras Shambra, on the coast of northern Syria,
13 B.C.; Mami was perhaps ambassador or even viceroy of the king of Egypt.)
(b) Simplified cross section of the relief with unworked intermediate space; compare with figure 7b.

6. GESTALT LAWS

Now why is it that, among the variously colored stimulated areas that
adjoin one another in the eye, usually without our having any part in
it, one area in particular becomes a formed figure, and the other formless
ground?

It is not always as simple as with the outline of the sky, for which
you know in advance that the sky is not an object, but actually continues
behind foreground objects. There are plenty of cases in which one cannot know anything about a bounded area in advance, or on the contrary

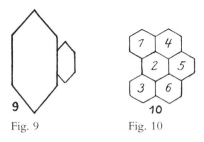

Fig. 9   Fig. 10

Figure 9
Only the common part of the two hexagons is a boundary to both sides.

Figure 10
Honeycomb figure. Every interior line is a boundary to both sides. If one asks mentally retarded pupils to continue this pattern in the proper sequence, drawings such as in figures 11a,b, and d result.

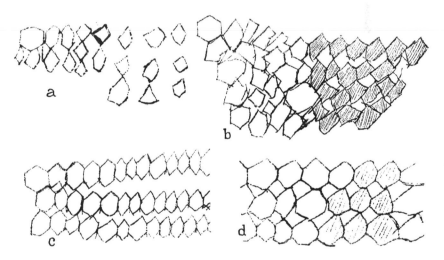

Figure 11
(a) and (b) The most backward pupils draw only lines that bound unilaterally; hatching inside the cells was added later to make this more salient. (c) At least the vertical lines have become bilateral boundaries, but only because the prescribed sequence was not followed. (d) Real progress: only small line segments at the intersections remain unilateral boundaries. (From H. Rupp: *Über optische Analyse. Psychol. Forschg.* 4, 1923.)

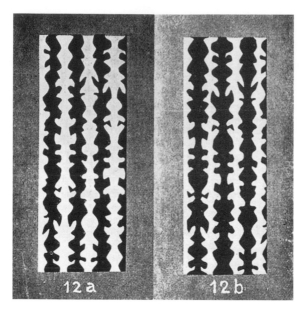

Figure 12
The role of the balance of form [symmetry]. Usually on the left (a) one sees white, on the right (b) black figures, i.e., always the balanced [symmetrical] parts of the field. (After P. Bahnsen: *Symmetrie und Asymmetrie bei visuellen Wahrnehmungen. Z. Psychol.* 108, 1928.)

one knows for sure that there really is nothing behind it. In the case of a mosaic ornament with, let us say a gold pattern on a blue ground, everybody knows that the gold and blue tiles lie peacefully next to each other and that there is nothing behind them but cement. Nevertheless the golden parts appear to lie shaped on top of the blue ones that formlessly continue underneath them. Why does the blue, conversely, not appear to lie on the gold, even when the golden parts are newly invented shapes rather than familiar objects (flowers and the like)?

Closer scrutiny reveals a remarkable set of psychological laws that have been called *Gestalt laws*. We see a particularly important law, the *law of closure*, active in figure 2. We have drawn the dark intermediate spaces completely enclosed, whereas the light letters at top and bottom are left open, but the spaces that are closed have a better chance of appearing as a formed figure than the open ones. In figure 3 the law of *symmetry* comes into play, among others. The black part has a symmetrical structure, whereas the two flanking white parts, taken individually, do not; the symmetrical form is balanced in itself, and thus has a

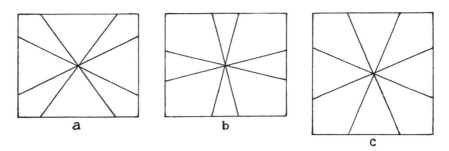

Figure 13
The role of narrow and wide (near and far). (a) one usually sees a diagonal cross, in (b) an upright cross with (c) an unstable alternating percept, since all fields are equal in width.

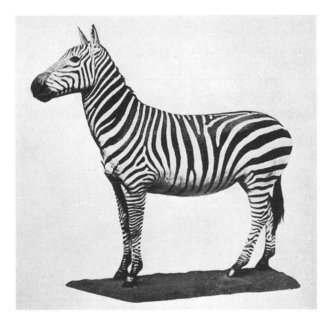

Figure 14
The zebra: is it white with black stripes or black with white ones?

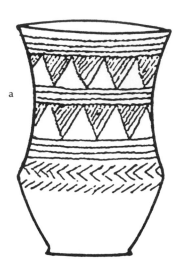

a

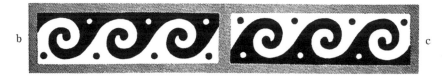

b   c

Figure 15

Reversing patterns. (a) Neolithic beaker from the age of string pottery at the end of the Neolithic period, Holzheim, District Gießen. (From A. van Scheltema: *Die alt-nordische Kunst*. Berlin, 1924.) Are these light upright triangles or dark inverted ones? (b) and (c) Old Greek wave band (After W. Ehrenstein: *Untersuchungen über Figur-Grundfragen. Z. Psychol*. 117, 1930.) (b) Is this a white pattern that points upward or a black one that points down? (c) The same pattern inverted: black upward or white downward?

greater likelihood of appearing as a formed figure than the asymmetrical ones (figure 12).

Another important law is the law of *proximity*. Each of the three panels of figure 13 has eight adjacent areas. But initially you do not see all eight. In (a) you see a slanted cross, in (b) one that stands upright: the narrower parts become "things" (arms of the cross), the wider parts become intermediate spaces. But here the figure is so simple that with an effort you can see a very broad upright cross with narrow intermediate spaces in (a) or a tilted one in (b). Proximity and closure work together in the case of small openings, especially when they occur in large, regu-lar surfaces, for example a keyhole. That is why you can see the shape of

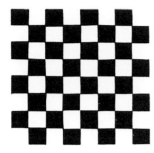

Figure 16
Checkerboard pattern, the simplest and most disturbing reversible pattern. The Greeks of the classical period rejected this pattern in weaving as "barbaric." (Cf. also p. 43.)

a keyhole even though it is really a kind of intermediate space. The law of proximity played a role in our mysterious inscription (figure 2) as well: we also drew the dark parts narrower than the lighter ones, otherwise they would have become figures much less easily despite their closure.

7. Reversible Patterns

If none of the Gestalt laws is decisive (figure 13c), the figure vacillates back and forth between the upright and the slanted cross and never comes to rest. All of a sudden what was just figure becomes background, and vice versa. People who are particularly sensitive can be driven crazy by such reversible patterns. Fortunately for our peace of mind, reversible patterns rarely occur in natural environments: the zebra (figure 14) is one of the few creatures that frequently is drawn in such a way that you can annoy your friends by asking them whether it really is white with black stripes or black with white stripes. The confusing stimulus of this ambiguous pattern (figures 15a–c) was discovered as early as the end of the Neolithic period. When you see carpet, tile, or wallpaper patterns that drive you crazy, it is often—not always—because the patterns are reversible, as in figure 13c. The simplest example is the common checkerboard pattern that only sturdy people can tolerate for an extended period of time (figure 16).

The invisibility of the shape of intermediate spaces or of parts of the ground is one of the most important techniques used in puzzle pictures. Indeed, our figures 2 and 3 are just like a kind of puzzle picture reduced to an especially simple form for clarity. We did not have to turn the figure in question upside down or to hide it with extra branch lines and cross-hatching. It stands there upright and exposed, and yet it remains invisible to the naive observer.

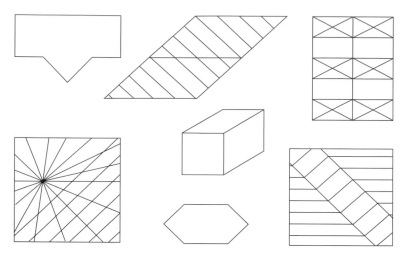

Figure 16A

Invisible shapes. The diagram contains three identical hexagons, three identical squared blocks, and three identical rectangles with a point (as above left). Where are they? How long did the search take? Who can see all of them without the help of a pencil or laboriously gathering up their parts over and over? (From K. Gottschaldt: *Über den Einfluß der Erfahrung* etc. *Psychol. Forschg.* 8, 1926.)

Figure 16A provides a natural transition to chapter 2, which deals with invisible figures of a different kind.

2

Visible and Invisible Forms

1. Natural and Artificial Parts: The Hidden Ambiguity of Everything Seen

We begin with an experiment: On a piece of paper we draw two equal, intersecting circles of approximately 10 cm diameter (figure 17), place a piece of blotting paper underneath and punch out the circles with a pencil. On the backside of the paper we then have the image in "Braille." Now we let an assistant (preferably a schoolchild) feel this image with eyes blindfolded, without having shown it to him before, and then request, after the image and the blindfold are removed, that it be drawn from memory. The result is often an unexpected image, such as the outline of a bread roll with an almond in it (figure 18a). At first you might think: "but that's wrong, he didn't notice that it is two circles." You may well reflect on the imperfection of the sense of touch, until you suddenly realize that the sense of touch has made a discovery here that the eyes could not easily see.

The drawing (figure 18a) is also correct and there are many other versions that would be correct, for example, two sickles (figure 18b) or four open arcs (figure 19a), or one continuous line that can resemble a pretzel, among other things (figure 19b). Quite aside from the intermediate spaces,[4] countless other shapes are always present before our eyes *that we cannot see in the least.* Among these are always some shapes that are very familiar to us, or at least more familiar than those that become "visible." Where we see three rather unusual stretches of lines, one jagged, one wavy, and one irregularly circular, some shapes can also be hidden, for example, the familiar numeral "4" (figure 20).

For us readily to see a form, it must belong to a part of the visual field that *holds together in itself and is sharply delineated against what is around*

---

4. See p. 3 section 3.

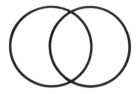

Figure 17
Two intersecting circles; or perhaps something else? See figure 18. (Figures 17–19 from Becker: *Über taktil-motorische Figurwahrnehmung. Psychol. Forschg.* 20, 1934.)

Figure 18
Two more possible ways to see figure 17. (a) The sense of touch teaches us that figure 17 actually can also be something else: a "mantle" in the form of a bread roll and a "core" in the form of an almond. (b) Another possibility one does not think of immediately: the figure could also be the image of two sickles [crescents].

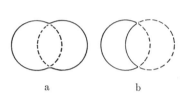

a   b

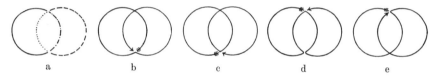

a   b   c   d   e

Figure 19
Some more possibilities to structure figure 17: how do we know that it is not four open arcs (a)? Or a somewhat bent pretzel (b)? Or a "3" that has become somewhat portly, lying down (c)? Or an oddly curved kind of Latin "W" (d)? Or a badly twisted "8" (e)? But only the articulation into two circles seems to us to be correct.

it. If these two conditions are not met, we are just as blind to the shapes in question as to the in-between spaces. The sorts of shapes that happen to be visible therefore depend completely on the *articulations* of what is seen: In order to be able to see the "4" in figure 20, one must first mentally cut through each of the three continuous lines twice and join the two cut-off ends anew into an angle at one of the intersections.

The effort required for that unnatural segmentation demonstrates that it is in *no way a voluntary choice* as to what gets organized together in perception. The old view too, that things always appear to belong together that in our experience have most often appeared together, cannot be right, for in this case they are doubtless the parts of the "4." If the articulation of what is seen were left entirely to chance, then for example, if three people were to look at figure 17, the first might see two circles, the second two sickles, and the third the forms of a roll with an almond, and any additional person might see something else; mutual un-

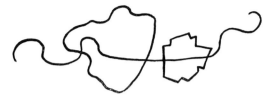

Figure 20
A new puzzle picture. It contains a meaningful and familiar shape; which is it? The numeral 4! Here an explanation from experience fails, because everybody surely knows a 4 better than three strange continuous lines. (Figures 20–22 after Köhler: *Psychologische Probleme*. Berlin, 1933.)

derstanding would not at all be possible. Thus there must be *underlying laws* of perceptual organization according to which everything seen is organized, laws that are generally universal across individuals. The shapes that spontaneously emerge according to these laws without our interference, and that we find complete (for example, the two circles in figure 17), contrasted with the later found or unnaturally contrived alternative articulations (figures 18 and 19), give the incontrovertible impression of being the "genuine," "true," "natural" parts.

Nevertheless it is wrong to believe that the "natural" organization is fully determined by the configuration of the stimuli in the eye; because, as we found, the stimulus configuration is extraordinarily ambiguous,[5] even though we may not be aware of that ambiguity. A closer examination of the relationships at that decisive location, at the stimulated sensory surface in the eye, reveals that the natural organization holds not even the slightest advantage over alternative organizations based on the stimulus distribution. That advantage must be due, therefore, to the *laws of vision* themselves, according to which everything seen organizes itself and thereby also receives its form. It is on these laws that we wish to focus.

2.   THE LAW OF THE SMOOTHLY CONTINUOUS CURVE: THE BREAK AS A BORDER

No naïve observer would readily discern in figure 21 the parts shown in figure 22. Even when it is no longer contested that those parts really are

---

5. We will see later that this is true for every stimulus configuration, even the simplest (see p. 38 section 5).

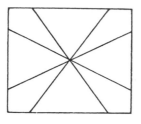

Figure 21
Rectangle with cross; but now we naturally suspect that
all sorts of other things lie hidden in it.

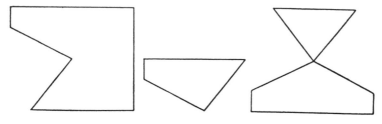

Figure 22
Parts also contained in figure 21, but which a naive observer never sees, because lines
at an angle are continued in places where in figure 21 a straight, smooth continuation
would also be possible.

contained within it, just as much as the rectangle and the slanted cross,
nevertheless something in them does not seem right, as with the parts in
figures 18 and 19. Again and again the lines are continued at an angle in
places where straight (figure 21) or gradually curved (figure 17) continuations would also be possible. Parts of a curve that run into each
other at an "angle" of 180 degrees are generally compellingly seen as
unstructured units. It is not easy for anyone to see figure 23a as two
drops touching each other, or figure 23b as a "hexagon with two collapsed corners," even though there is no geometric objection to these
interpretations. Only where there is no straight (or otherwise smooth)
continuation at the corners does a break occur by itself. There is therefore always only one line that ends at a *"branch point,"* and *none at all at*
"line crossings."

However, the crossings and branchings are not quite without consequences even for smoothly continuous curves. Natural and artificial
new boundaries occur exclusively at such characteristic places (figures
18, 19, 22, and 23). You could imagine yet other, quite different new
structures; for example, with the pair of rings (figure 17), the division
into a cross, two angular pieces, and nine different large pieces of an arc
(figure 24), as if a shattered pair of glass rings were brought together

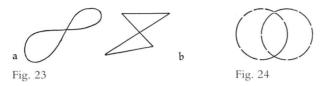

Fig. 23   Fig. 24

Figure 23
A bow-tie (a) and a quadrilateral that crosses over itself (b); usually one does not notice that the one could be a pair of drops and the other a hexagon with two collapsed corners. The reason is the same as with figure 22.

Figure 24
Even a cross (lower center), two angled V-pieces touching point-to-point (upper center), and nine irregular arc segments, are legitimate "parts" of figure 17, for it could be decomposed in that way. Similarly, one could also think up 1,000 other divisions or cut them out with scissors. But when there are no breaks or cuts in the figure then, we generally cannot see them.

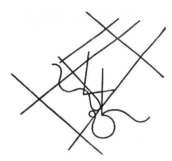

Figure 25
Might the unfamiliar surround be the reason that one does not immediately see the "4" in figure 20? No, because here the surround is certainly just as unfamiliar and nonetheless the numeral pops out clearly. (From Köhler: *Psychologische Probleme.* Berlin, 1933.)

again and reconstructed out of its fragments. But you cannot see this (like the division into two sickles) as long as there are no breaks (figure 24). You also cannot see that every triangle could also represent a quadrilateral with one angle of 180 degrees even when you consider the matter geometrically, in which case this must be treated as a transition case. Now we already know the most important reason why the numeral 4 is not perceived in figure 20, but is readily perceived in figure 25, even though the additions in the latter are just as unusual as in the former.

3. THE LAW OF THE GOOD GESTALT: THE LOVE OF ORDER OF OUR SENSES

We now know why figure 21 appears to be composed of eight straight lines. But why does one see these lines as a diagonal cross and a frame,

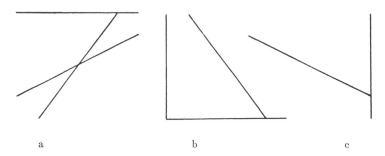

a   b   c

Figure 26
Three parts out of which figure 21 can be put together correctly. With this division, no straight line is cut through. Nevertheless one can only see these three parts with great difficulty in figure 21, because in comparison with the cross and the rectangle they are crooked and disorderly.

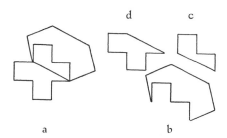

Figure 27
(a) Cross and hexagon; or what else? (b–d) One could just as readily see figure 27(a) divided into these pieces, if only our eyes were not so fond of order.

instead of just as easily as three groups as in figure 26? Instead of the Greek cross and the hexagon (figure 27a), why does one not see just as easily three surface areas lying next to each other (figures 27b–d)? Why, instead of the straight and the S line (figure 28a) do we not just as readily perceive two walking sticks (figure 28b and c)? In figures 26, 27b, c, and d, and 28b and c, the law of good continuation is not violated anywhere. But compared with the "natural" divisions—Maltese cross and rectangle (figure 21), Greek cross and hexagon (figure 27a), straight line and S curve—these part configurations are irregular, crooked, and disorganized in structure. There are often prominent irregularities and these are *only of limited stability* in perception. When the stimulus distribution (as in figures 21, 27a, and 28b) permits an organization in simple, orderly, Gestalten constructed according to a unitary rule, then these "good" or prägnant forms prevail.

The law of *balanced form*, or law of symmetry, which we found in the previous section, is only a special case—although a particularly ef-

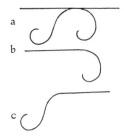

a

b

c

Figure 28

(a) A straight line and an S curve; but compare figures 28(b) and (c): two hooked canes; parts we normally do not see in figure 28a, even though they are just as smooth as the straight line and the S, which prevail because of their still greater unity.

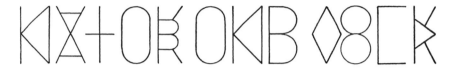

Figure 29

Another mysterious inscription

their shape is exactly as usual.

until one covers the upper half. Over each letter is its mirror image. According to laws of symmetry and proximity, the lines become organized more strongly verti-cally than to the left or right; the laws of the smooth curve and of closure work in the same way. Thus, for the naïve observer the letters are unrecognizable, although

fective one—of this general law. To get to know its unifying power, one could place a piece of unframed mirror glass with a straight edge directly on the upper border of a written or printed line (figure 29). Almost irresistibly each letter fuses with its mirror image in front of our eyes, so that even in this larger context and in the usual environment the letters, which one has read countless times before, are harder to see than the mostly unfamiliar mirror-image structures.[6]

Particularly hard to make out in figure 29 are the U and the V, also the N. Here the law of *good continuation* and particularly the law of *closure*, which we also met earlier,[7] and which are also special cases of the general law of order or *prägnanz* come into play. The same law is active when, while searching for invisible parts (for example from figures 17 and 27), you find first closed figures, figures in which the lines form the perimeter of a surface area (figures 18 and 22); and only later and with more difficulty do we notice those that consist of open (figure

6. With bridges, planks, trees, and posts near or in mirror-calm water the fusion of the mirror image often occurs just as convincingly as here despite all our experience.

7. See p. 10.

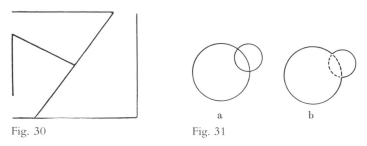

Fig. 30   Fig. 31

Figure 30

A particularly senseless and therefore hard-to-find part of figure 21. It simultaneously violates the Gestalt laws of the smooth curve, closure, and symmetry. If one
tries to memorize and force it to be seen in figure 21, it still slips away again and
again.

Figure 31

Two unequal circles (a); here even when feeling a tactile stimulus, one no longer
perceives the "kernel and mantle" (b) as in figure 18a. For kernel and mantle are no
longer double mirror-symmetric and also no longer have a common center. Even
the tactile sense is sensitive to the unusual regularity. (After Becker; see figure 17.)

19a), intertwined (figures 19b–e), or branching (figures 26 and 30) line
segments.

It is also important that the individual structural parts of the image
stand in a mutually orderly relationship. This is the case, for example,
when the seen object is structured into parts with a common center
and common axes of symmetry. From this law of the *common center* it
becomes understandable why the pair of circles (figure 17) can also naturally become structured into an almond in a surrounding roll, at least
when using the tactile sense (figure 18). You only need to eliminate the
aforementioned factors (figure 31a) and the structure still organizes itself
only into two circles, even through touch alone. The almond-in-a-roll
organization would now be just as "disorderly" as perhaps for figure 27
(cf. figure 32).

Even in cases where a smooth continuation would be possible, one
nevertheless sees angular units, if in this way the structure of the parts
becomes more unitary (figure 33 and especially figure 34). It is precisely
that which naturally "belongs together" that gets organized together.
And what belongs together is that which "fits" together; that is, that
which together results in a well-organized, unitary structure. Things that
by virtue of their chance position appear to belong to something else as
a necessary component can in this way disappear from our view, even

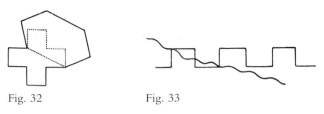

Fig. 32   Fig. 33

Figure 32
Such deformities would arise if figure 27 were seen as structured according to the pattern of figure 18 into kernel and mantle.

Figure 33
Wavy line and crenellated line. The preference for the greatest unity in the whole contradicts in two places the preference for a smooth continuation. Here, the structure arranges itself according to the greatest unity in the whole. (From Wertheimer: *Untersuchungen zur Lehre von der Gestalt. Psychol. Forschg.* 4, 1923.)

Figure 34
Zigzag line and octagon. The opposition of two different figural preferences, as in figure 33, with that preference dominating that includes the larger field. If one draws on an empty sheet of paper first the line in the direction of the arrow, and then one after the other adds the other lines, one can clearly see how finally the straight line is cut up.

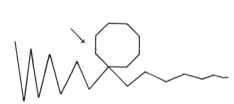

though they are lying completely exposed. You can make a nice party game out of openly hiding erasers, pencils, and other things up to the size of a walking stick (figure 35) by using the law of intermediate space described above.

Figures that are unified in the larger context do not always exhibit the smoothest component lines and curves. But those that have both global unity and smooth component curves create emergent structural organizations that are especially robust, and, at the same time the less smooth and regular organizations disappear so thoroughly (figure 36) that all crossing out (figure 37) in comparison is clumsy. To be sure, you can understand this lawfulness only when you consider the whole: the hidden hexagon considered by itself is not much less regular than most of the figures which you see naturally in figure 36. But if you consider what sorts of deformed figures would have to emerge aside from

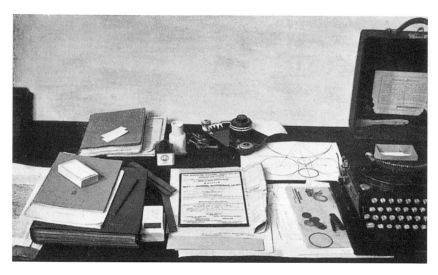

Figure 35

"Enchanted room" according to the law of Gestalt belongingness: Things lying in the open that seem to be an essential component of a larger whole are much harder to find than things that by chance all by themselves lie between or on top of other things. One of the two long pencils outlines a side of the black funerary edge; the one small rubber band lies on the geometric drawing as if the drawing were incomplete without it; the coin acts as if it were one of the keys of the typewriter; the stopper of the black bottle crowns the ink pot as if it had never done anything else; two of the four small cards look like adhesive labels belonging to the small pen case.

the hidden figure if it became segregated (figure 38), it is no longer surprising that this organization does not tend to appear. If the accompanying lines are so arranged that they together create a halfway orderly figure, preferably with a common center of gravity (figure 39b), the hidden figure can then at least be easily discerned despite the straight sides of the triangle and despite the greater simplicity of the triangles (figure 39a).

Many unitary wholes consist purely of equal parts; but this too does not have to be so. In figure 34, the lower half of the straight line fuses perceptually with many lines of different lengths and orientations into a zigzag, even though all the sides of the octagon are exactly the same size and some are also oriented the same way.

In general, one must not form too narrow a concept of the term "good Gestalt." Granted that it includes such simple forms as a straight line, a circle, and a square, for which one can immediately specify a geometric or algebraic formula that stands out through its simplicity. But countless other shapes that are not so easy to specify mathematically also

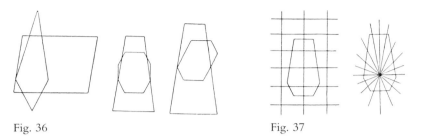

Fig. 36   Fig. 37

Figure 36

Three simple puzzle pictures which each contain the same irregular hexagon as in figure 37. But here the law of the smooth curve and the law of the good Gestalt work together to create a different kind of organization. The hexagon is thus so thoroughly hidden that one must trace it in order not to lose sight of it. (From Wertheimer: *Untersuchungen zur Lehre von der Gestalt. Psychol. Forschg.* 4, 1923.)

Figure 37

The hexagon is crossed out; many more lines pass across it than in figure 36. Nevertheless it remains clearly visible. According to Gestalt laws (see text) both the hexagon and the additional lines each make up a group by themselves without our assistance.

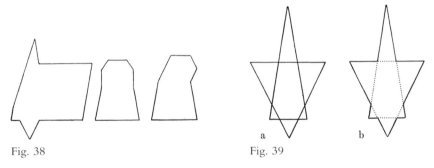

Fig. 38   Fig. 39

Figure 38

Such irregular shapes would tend to appear instead of the hexagon, if it were to segregate itself in figure 36; it does not help much that the hexagon itself has a reasonably regular form.

Figure 39

All sides of the hexagon continue straight, and two much simpler figures arise: triangles (a). Nevertheless the hexagon is easy to find, for now the remaining figure is tolerably formed. A somewhat irregular star (b), and also the hexagon is the core now sitting nicely in the middle, like the kernel in figure 18.

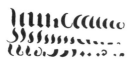

Figure 40
Components of German printed script (Gothic style). They are much more numerous and much less simple than in Roman script. Nevertheless one can read the German printed script more effortlessly. It does not depend on the shape of the components, not even on the shape of individual letters, but only on the shape of the whole words, and this can be more legible with tangled components than with simple ones. (From Saudek: *Experimentelle Graphologie.*)

exhibit good Gestalt, namely, all those shapes that give the impression that this is "harmonious, from one stroke," starting with the often difficult-to-specify *tension* and *streaming* forms, up to the incalculable shapes of higher animals. It also holds true for these kinds of good Gestalt that, in the organization of what is seen, they dominate "poorer," "arbitrary," or "piecemeal" shapes as far as the distribution of the stimulus permits.

The unfortunate and failed battle against the German, or Gothic, font in favor of the Roman script, which excited well-meaning souls for a while, rested on the erroneous proposition that a good and therefore easily recognizable shape is only one that is composed entirely of simple components; and simple components, from the same error, were understood to be those that could be constructed with ruler and compass. The components of German printed script were displayed in tables, in order to show convincingly how unnecessarily numerous and ridiculously tangled they are, especially in the capitals (figure 40). Careful experiments, however, showed that the general overview of printed lines, which is all that counts, was never worse with the German script, and often was better than with the Roman (compare the study by Rudolph Schwegmann, Göttingen 1935.) [Translators' note: the Roman script won out in the end, and is now the standard for the German language, although this may have been more for compatibility with other European languages than for any intrinsic merits of the Roman font.]

Thus one could say in a somewhat facetious way that even the most disorderly human being has at least, without realizing it, *eyes that love order.* Otherwise, as shown in our examples, we would see the world filled with unthinkable deformities. But recall what awkward thoughts and artificial constructs were required in order to discover some of these alternative, less regular relations, and what an effort was required just to *see* them! If we open our eyes without any other intention than to see what is there, then among all the possible organizations of what is presented, our experience is the most perfect or regular interpretation that is possible at that moment. Our efforts arbitrarily to impose a less orderly interpretation are met with the strongest, often invincible, resistance. And the other higher senses—hearing, touch, sense of movement—behave just the same in their respective areas.

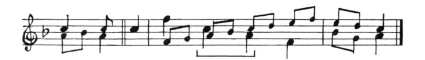

The generalization of the Gestalt laws of visual grouping into other sensory modalities is often quite remarkable. If two violins play the notes before the double bar, then following the law of good continuation the two Cs combine to form the upper voice and the sequence A-B-A becomes the lower voice. However, if the same tones are in the second, longer sequence,[8] then that is grouped together perceptually, as in figure 34, which in the broader context yields the more unitary wholes: the linear development C-C is cut apart: the first A and the B together with the second C form a part of an ascending scale in eighth-notes, while the first C joins the second A in a descending triad in quarter notes, irrespective of whether the violinists divide the voices in this or another way between them. When more voices with a similar sound are added, the tone group usually organizes itself again into an upper and a lower boundary voice with filling tones in between, which have primarily a coloring effect and are only loosely or not at all linked with the continuous melody; one hears "multiple sounds." The impression of a web of voices now arises only if other Gestalt laws cooperate: the law of proximity and especially the law of similarity (p. 32); that is, when, for example, the bass or a wind player takes over the third voice. That is why the structure of many-voiced canons and fugues becomes blurred when they are performed with only women's voices or only string players. In order to permit the composer's intent to emerge, such works must be performed on instruments with different sounds. Not every Gestalt law can be transferred unmodified to hearing, for instance not the law of closure and even less so the law of symmetry. We will return to circumstances in the sense of touch later.

---

8. Gluck, Sonata a tre no. 6 in F major, beginning of second movement.

3

Of Groups and Borders

1. Again the Law of Proximity

Why on a printed page do we see words, not just individual letters, even though the letters are not connected? The usual answer is: we have learned that these letters have meaning in a certain combination, and we see this combination. To test this answer, let us try using letter combinations alone to determine the meaning of a text. As you can see in the following few lines: *thelettersstillgroupintofamiliarwordswhenthespacesbetween themareentirelyabsentbutreadinghasbecomemuchharder*. We can also test which is more important for grasping the words, the meaning or the in-between space, *asi fasi napop ularch ild ren' sgam eweag ainint roduce largeri nters pace sbu twhe reac cordi ngtot hem eanin gtheyd ono tbel ong*. If one does not try hard, the in-between spaces determine the structural organization and one sees, despite all experience, strange, senseless syllables instead of well-known, meaningful words.

In meaningless collections of similar forms (figure 41), the effect of spacing dominates. You do not see six single spots, but two groups of them. And in the same way you see in the heavens not single stars, but stellar constellations, long before you are taught about them and learn their names. Aside from memorizing names, learning about constellations thus consists mostly of the addition of incidental appendages to existing constellation groupings, and in finding inconspicuous and thus far unnoticed new groups. The task of ignoring incorrectly formed false groups is only rarely necessary. The *law of proximity* thus determines not only what becomes a figure (p. 11), but quite often what ought to be grouped together in the first place. This perceptual grouping works just as well for a child today as for astronomers in antiquity, from whom we have taken most of the names of constellations. The same perceptual grouping holds for the astronomer of the present day, undiminished by his knowledge from his own measurements that the stars that seem to form a group actually lie worlds apart and have no real connection.

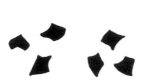

Figure 41
Not six patches, but twice three patches; neighbors fuse into groups. Other organizations, for example into three pairs, require effort and fall apart immediately when the effort subsides. (From W. Köhler: *Psychol. Probleme.* Berlin, 1933.)

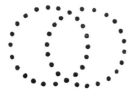

Figure 42
The dotted pair of circles is hardly different from the drawn one (figure 17, p. 16). There are not forty-two dots, but rather two circles with dots on them. Gestalt laws work unchanged despite partition and interruption.

2. BRIDGING LINES AND IMAGINED LINES

The fusion of spatially separated objects in perception is associated with a curious change in the spaces between them. What happens when you present a pair of intersecting circles (figure 42) using dots instead of lines? Instead of uninterrupted black lines, there are forty-two dots. Although they are located along the former curves, the smoothness of the curves, one might say, is destroyed by dozens of wide gaps. Nevertheless this change means almost nothing! As before, one sees two rings with dots on them. Often in such cases one cannot remember afterward whether one saw the figure drawn continuously or dotted. The short distances across which the fusion occurs are different from the large gaps that are empty all across. They become a type of *bridge*. And these bridges are all the more striking, the smaller the scale of the group and the more delicate the coloring of the parts. If you pencil a couple of fine, barely visible dots some 2 to 5 mm apart on a piece of paper, you begin to wonder whether there may not perhaps be real connecting lines there (paper fibers, etc.). Someone who has not seen the drawing being produced could hardly tell whether or not the connecting lines are also drawn. The fact that it is a matter of bridging lines becomes clear if you displace the dots, which in turn displaces the perceived line. The once so famous and mysterious canals on Mars (figure 42A) were also illusory conjunctions of this type. The same Gestalt laws apply to bridging lines as for real lines: figure 42 illustrates the laws of good continuation, of simplicity, of closure, and, in the tactile sense, that of a common center; these too, like any other lines, can also become the edges of figural surfaces and the like.

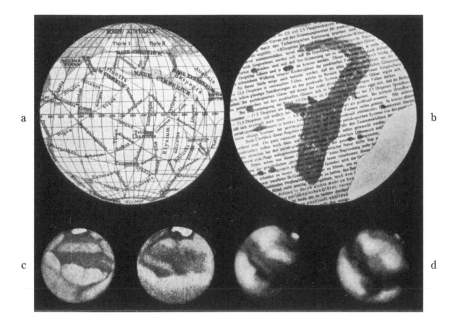

Figure 42A

The planet Mars (a) from a map by Schiaparelli (1888). (b) "Mars" made with news-print; with suitable illumination (squint!) and viewing distance, "canals" run from the ledges to the dots and between them (From A. Kuhl: *Vjschr. Astron. Ges.* 59, 1924). (c, d) Also in newer drawings there is more to be seen than on the best photograph, nonetheless not much is left of the canals.

But is it not a little presumptuous to assert that we actually see the bridging lines? Are these not simply imaginary lines, as used daily by the mathematician? This doubt is easily dispelled. You can place an imaginary line wherever you choose, but not a bridging line. In a dotted circle you can easily think, for example, of two points on opposite sides of the circle as connected by an imaginary diameter. But you cannot see all the imagined diameters of the circle simultaneously, as you see the bridging lines on the circumference. If dots are arranged in a regular polygon (figure 43), then the bridging lines appear as straight line segments, up to about the octagon. For dot polygons with more than ten vertices, the bridging lines are clearly curved and closed, forming a circle, although you can still imagine straight connecting lines. If you draw arbitrary bridging lines (figure 44) next to some natural bridging lines in a well-known grouping of dots, the group is no longer recognizable. But if only the bridging lines are drawn (figure 45A), then there is no essential difference between the drawing and the actual group of dots (figure

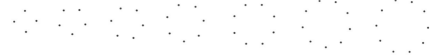

Figure 43

Regular polygons from dots. Up to an octagon, the bridging lines are straight and form a polygon. After that they become curved and form a circle, although we can still imagine straight connections. Bridging lines and imagined lines are therefore not the same. (From Koffka: *Psychol. d. opt. Wahrnehmg*, in Bethe's *Hdb. d. Physiol.* 12, Section 2.)

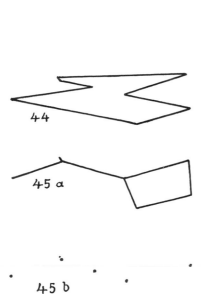

Figure 44

What is this? No one recognizes in this image the constellation of the Big Dipper, although the corner points correspond exactly. The natural bridging lines are replaced in part by arbitrary connections. (From M. Hertz: *Das optische Gestaltproblem und der Tierversuch. Verh. Dtsch. Zool. Ges.* 1929.)

Figure 45

The Big Dipper. If you draw only the natural bridging lines (a), then the constellation (b) hardly seems to be changed: the lines were actually already there, but not emphasized in this way.

45b). This means that in the latter drawing (figure 45A) new lines have not been added to the dots, but rather the lines that really were already present in the perceptual image, have only, so to speak, been *emphasized.*

3. THE LAW OF SIMILARITY

When the two natural groups of figure 41 are not separated too far and are not too dense, we can easily break them apart. We need only, for example, color the three upper spots red, reduce them in size, make them ring-shaped or cross-hatch them, and so on, and we easily get two

Figure 46
The law of similarity in competition with the law of proximity. Proximity requires
three left, three right; similarity requires three above, three below.

new groups that now extend over the longer distance (figure 46). Especially strong is the effect of equal color. So there is an organizational law
of *similarity*. Similarity strives toward unification, even across considerable interspaces. Similar parts result in more unitary, purer groups than
dissimilar ones. The law of similarity is thus again a special case of the
general law of the *unity of structure*, or of the law of the *good Gestalt*.[9]
Total identity binds together best. If there are no identical items, the
most similar ones or those that otherwise result in an especially unitary whole are organized together, for example, a uniform brightness
staircase.

But what appears equal or similar depends again itself on the
circumstances. A difference, which by itself leads to the formation of a
clear border, can become ineffective when a significantly stronger difference occurs in the region (figure 47), so that the image that was previously segregated from the background now disappears. A housewife
uses this law when she chooses for her house-dress, or the rug in the
children's room, a fabric that is as strongly patterned as possible.[10] The
same law prevails that when looking through open windows in a bright
house wall, you see largely nothing but uniform darkness, even though
there is daylight in the room.[11] Glare, in the narrowest sense—such
as from the headlights of an oncoming car—is just an especially pro-
nounced effect of this kind. This effect is also seen clearly around a distant street lamp. If the view of the lamp itself it blocked with a narrow

9. See p. 19 section 3.

10. When the pattern consists of small dots or spots, the effect of Gestalt "belongingness" is added, according to which even distinctly segregated spots of dirt become
invisible, so that it looks as though they belonged to the pattern; compare p. 24,
figure 35.

11. The well-known *law of contrast* implies for this case only that within the brighter
surround of the house exterior wall, objects in the interior of the room would look
too dark, but not that they would also become totally indistinguishable. This holds
also for the further examples of true glare.

a

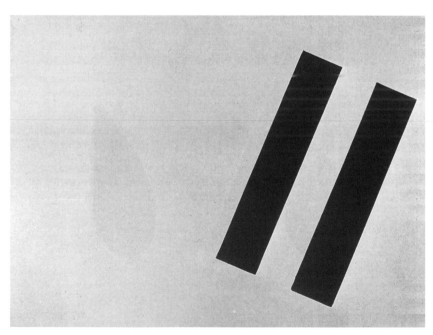

b

black band that occludes the light source, it is astounding how much
more can suddenly be seen around it. Here are significant and thus far
hardly used opportunities to increase safety on nocturnal streets. As we
will see later, the law of suppression of small contrasts by larger ones
also plays an important role in animate nature.

An example of similarity that has a particularly striking organizing
effect is the law of *common fate*. If you glue three patches each (from figure 41) made of dark paper on two identical sheets of glass, perhaps the
upper spots on one, the lower spots on the other, and then superimpose
the glass sheets and observe them against the light (or make them cast
shadows against the wall), you see the two original groups fall apart and
both horizontal rows merge together as soon as the two glass panes are
moved relative to each other. By the same principle, flickering flames
in a row of lanterns seem to be in a mysterious connection, even when
they are not next to each other; just as a barely noticeable wisp of a
breeze can magically reveal the outline of an aspen out of the leaves
rustling at the edge of the forest. Here too the effect is particularly compelling when all the parts move in synchrony, as in our experiment
above, as well as when you see a solid body move coherently against
a background. But the connection—and the relevant figure-ground
segregation—even occurs when local motions are not entirely identical.
If three flies sit still on a window pane and three others crawl around on
it, the three that are moving seem to belong together, even if they are
moving in different directions. For this reason it is also wrong to believe
that the law of common fate involves only a matter of memory of the
known behavior of solid bodies.

4. A FEW MORE APPLICATIONS OF GESTALT LAWS

One of the most striking applications of structural laws that have been
discussed is the sewing cut-out pattern, in which a great number of large

◀ **Figure 47**
The large color difference weakens or destroys the boundary effect of the smaller
one. In (a) and (b) the exact same pair of spots is presented, but in (b) two black
bars are added to the finished print. In (a) both spots are approximately equally visible. In (b), the right spot has disappeared; you have to look carefully to discover
traces of it between the two bars. The fact that it is so hard to protect uniformly colored fabrics from stains is often (not always) because of the law of seeing illustrated
here. At the same time the figure teaches us that one can be blinded not just by light,
but also by darkness.

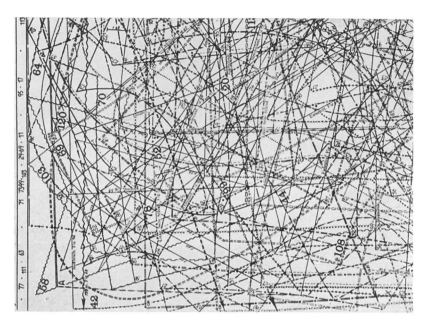

Figure 48
Piece of a sewing cut-out pattern. The fact that one can find one's way in the thick tangle of lines without practice depends on the artful use of the important laws of seeing (of similarity, of the smoothly continuous curve, of proximity, and of closure).

shapes must be accommodated on a restricted surface without producing any false connections (figure 48). The laws of similarity, proximity, good continuation, and, sometimes, closure are active here.

You can also observe the effects of consideration and neglect of Gestalt laws in written and printed communications of all kinds. An example is the inept handwriting [in older German script] with short connecting strokes between wide letters, in which one reads *Tranpeter* (a meaningless word) instead of *Trompeter* ("trumpeter"), and *Greule* (another meaningless word) instead of *Ohreule* ("horned owl"; figure 49). And then there is the frugal typing style in which the dash and the hyphen are typed without spaces between them to save room, and as a consequence, instead of giving structure to the sentence, the two neighboring words are hideously clumped together. One often finds poorly structured tables in which main numbers are scattered unrecognizably among crowds of auxiliary numbers. Finally we note scientific papers in which a hundred pages appear without paragraphs or detectable chapter

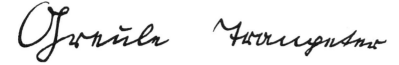

Figure 49

This older German handwriting should read *Ohreule* [horned owl] and *Trompeter* [trumpeter], but the law of proximity is not respected, so one reads "Greule" and "Tranpeter" [nonsense words].

> CUNCTAVIDENSMAGNOCURARUMFLUCTUATAESTU
> ADQUEANIMUMNUNCHUCCELEREMNUNCDIVIDITILLVC
> INPARTISQUERAPITUARIASPERQUEOMNIAVERSAT
> SICUTAQUAETREMULUMLABRISUBILUMENAENIS
> SOLEREPERCUSSUMAUTRADIANTISLMAGINELUNAE
> OMNIAPERVOLITATLATELOCAIAMQUESUBAURAS

Figure 50

A piece of a Latin manuscript probably from the 5th century C.E. (Vergil, *Aeneid*, 8th canto, Vatican Library) without spaces between words; only someone who knows the words can find their boundaries. The piece reads: . . . *cuncta videns magno curarum fluctuat aestu,* / *adque animum nunc huc celerem, nunc dividit illuc,* / *in partisque rapit varias perque omnia versat:* / *sicut aquae tremulum labris ubi lumen aenis* / *sole repercussum aut radiantis imagine lunae* / *omnia pervolitat late loca iamque sub auras* . . . (*Aeneid* VIII, 19–24), and means roughly: ". . . (when Aeneas) who saw the whole scene, tossed about in his trouble, wave after wave of it. He let his mind run this way and that, passing quickly over all he might do, like basins full of water, when struck by a ray of sunlight or the bright disk of the moon, a flickering light plays over walls and corners, flying up to hit high roof beams (and a coffered ceiling)."

headings, and in which important related findings, on whose direct comparison the entire investigation depends, are presented many pages apart.

Presumably, with newly invented scripts one is tempted to rely predominantly on the binding and separating effect of fixed and learned meanings. The ancient Greeks and Romans wrote without spaces between words (figure 50), like our lines 6 and 7 (p. 29). Only the cloistered scribes of the Middle Ages started intuitively to follow the laws of seeing in placing letters, and in so doing they advanced the art of reading almost as much as the inventor of the printing press. Significantly, the script most recently introduced in Europe, the abstract symbology of logic and discrete mathematics, has tentatively returned in some ways to the state of antiquity. Instead of the usual parentheses used in arithmetic—in which one can see directly from the curvature and mirror symmetry what is inside and what is out, and how far its inner part extends—it uses groups of dots, without insides or outsides, whose valid direction and extent must be sought out, like the beginnings of words and sentences in a 2,000-year-old manuscript. The two following formulas, whose content is irrelevant here, mean the same thing:

$$\vdash \; ::\text{p} \mid .\text{q} \mid \text{r}: \mid :.\text{t} \mid .\text{t} \mid \text{t}: \mid :\text{s} \mid \text{q}. \mid .\sim (\, \text{p} \mid \text{s} \,)$$

$$\vdash \left(\left\{ \text{p} \mid (\, \text{q} \mid \text{r} \,) \right\} \mid \left\{ \langle \text{t} \mid (\, \text{t} \mid \text{t} \,) \rangle \mid \langle [\, \text{s} \mid \text{q} \,] \mid [\sim (\, \text{p} \mid \text{s} \,)] \rangle \right\} \right)$$

If you cover up the bottom formula, you can immediately see how the upper one tends to decompose into a simple pattern of similar small-part groups. The logician, like the scribe in antiquity, will argue that with practice, the formula with the dots can be read, and this format saves work for the scribe. Although this is true, it also imposes a substantial burden on the reader. To find a truly economical symbology that combines the economy of the dots with the clarity of the parentheses, would be no trivial task.

5. THE MOST IMPORTANT APPLICATION IN NATURE: THE ABRUPT COLOR TRANSITION AS A BORDER

Let us look once more finally at our pair of circles[12] and make yet another new discovery: the fragments[13] are not even the most disorderly and unnatural arrangement you could think of for this drawing. You can, for example, tear the page with the drawing into scraps or shreds (figure 51). Or you send it by facsimile to a friend whereby the picture is sliced into many small shavings (figure 52) and then reassembled on the screen of the receiver set. In both cases you see, among other things, black and white parts. Or consider that the image in the eye is distributed in a punctiform raster across millions of tiny receptor cells, and on its way into the central nervous system is initially fragmented into nu-

---

12. See figure 17, p. 16.
13. See figure 24, p. 19.

Figure 51
Scraps or shreds. One can also divide the drawing of the two crossed rings in this manner, but only with the hands or in thought: in the intact drawing one can never see such parts.

Figure 52
Scan lines. Another unnatural division of our two rings; as is used in fax transmission [Translator's note: German "Bildfunk"], naturally using much finer slices. But one cannot see them in any case. (In the scan lines of the broadcast, the slanted borders between colored regions in each scan line are replaced by gradual transitions; but with the narrowness of the stripes this is not noticed in the reconstructed image.)

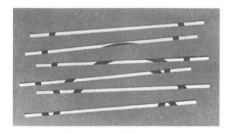

merous individual dots, none of which is apparent in the process of seeing (figure 53). We now know why it is impossible to see these divisions into scraps, shreds, or dots. Here the laws of similarity and proximity are working together, and thus both have the strongest possible effect. For the color of the entire paper and of the entire drawing is as similar as possible, namely, fully equal; and above all the distribution is as compact as possible, namely, without any differently colored space in between. Therefore, it is no wonder that in the inside of wider uniformly colored areas—apart from connecting lines—no boundaries can emerge, but rather only where differently colored areas immediately abut each other. The combined influence of these conditions also explains the (false!) impression that the unity of uniformly colored fields and the boundaries at abrupt color changes are propagated ready-made into our eyes.

The simultaneous action of similarity and immediate proximity described above is almost sufficient by itself to make perceived objects in our everyday environment organize themselves perceptually such that in most instances they correspond to our actual environment. For in nature self-contained objects (e.g., a stone) often consist of a uniform material or at least of a rather fine mixture, and for this reason they usually exhibit a rather uniform coloration, which contrasts with different, but again rather uniformly colored, neighboring objects (e.g., dirt or gravel); that is, it generates a boundary with them. The same is equally

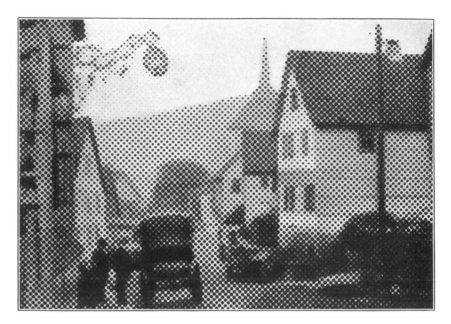

Figure 53

Pointillist; that is, a picture broken down into dots: a fully unnatural mode of division that one cannot see even with greatest effort, but that in perceptual theory has long played an undeserved role. In older texts you can still find the opinion that in reality one sees everything broken down into dots, and that in every case one needs to strain one's reason to figure out which dots belong together, and one's inventive talent to connect them together into familiar objects. The figure serves only for illustration; it is not a true representation of the relationships in the back of the eye. The screen in the retina of the eye—at least in its center—is honeycomb-like. (Illustration from *Natur und Volk*, 1931, p. 81.)

true for man-made tools and certainly for their major components when they are made out of a uniform material; and when not, they are usually colored intuitively according to natural rules of structure—unless, of course, the intent is to make them invisible; but more about that later.

It may now become clear why we have presented so many examples in which the eye fails in the absence of any kind of impairment. We are not doing this because of delight in the unusual. We have no time to dwell on peculiarities that arise only when one's sight is hindered—for example when one looks through a dirty window. Our goal is to investigate how the eye is capable of imparting useful information at all, given the great variety of shapes and things. Our question is: how must the eyes be configured so that the world looks neither like a swarm of countless independent and incoherent points of color, nor like a single sea of color in which everything is fused seamlessly with everything else? How is it that from our window on the world we do not see the 327 individual brightnesses and color tones that the painter must place upon the canvas in order to reproduce the view? Why do the 327 spots separate into precisely 3 entities of, for example, 120, 90, and 117 spots (i.e., into house, trees, and sky), instead of 2 entities of 150 and 177 spots or 7 entities of 6 times 50 and 27? And why precisely into these 3, and not rather into three others of perhaps 100 and 200 and 27?[14] The articulation of the perceived world into house, tree, and sky is especially adaptive for us living creatures; no other segmentation of the visual world would allow us to find our way so effortlessly around in our environment. But the utility of our perceptual representation does not explain anything, it rather deepens the mystery: because you don't often get something in this world just because you need it. The greatest thinkers have occupied themselves with this question without solving it. After Berkeley and Hume, the issue was addressed principally by Kant in the fundamental part of the *Critique of Pure Reason* entitled "Transcendental Analysis," especially in the second paragraph of the second major part *"On the a priori bases of the possibility of experience"* in which "experience" is intended to mean nothing other than information about things and events around us and in ourselves, regardless of how it comes to us. To find the proper answer to this question we must seek the limits of experience. We must attempt to determine at what point our senses begin to betray us, in the absence of the least bit of impairment or damage to the eye; at what point does the visual system no longer provide any discernable shape or structure in those cases where shapes are doubtless present. That is the only purpose and sense of the puzzle images we have discussed so far and that we will pursue further.

---

14. Compare Wertheimer: *Untersuchungen zur Lehre von der Gestalt*, II. *Psychol. Forschg.* 4, 1923.

4

Developmental Stages in Shape Formation

The stimulus distribution in the eye is *always infinitely ambiguous*. But only in rare cases does one notice this ambiguity without special reflection. The restlessness of the checkerboard pattern (figure 16) does not arise solely from the constant change between figure and ground. If one were to undertake to arrange it, as in figure 53A, as a black pattern on a white ground, its restlessness would be only slightly diminished. For it is impossible to see in such a pattern thirty-two independent squares or seventy-two independent dots. One senses how they try to order themselves into subdivisions: into left or right sloping, vertical or horizontal rows, upright or sloping rectangles, crosses, angles, and so on. But the different alternative organizations conflict and collide with each other so that they never settle into one coherent state. Nothing moves from its place and yet it is like an excited drill sergeant barking out his commands so fast that the troops do not know where they belong anymore. If the grid is not too large, the observer can sometimes create order at will: you simply decide to see a certain grouping, and that grouping actually appears. The success of such attempts to organize fluctuating perceptual groupings has occasionally led to the mistaken opinion that it is always attention, the direction of regard or gaze, in short, the behavior of the *observer* that structures the visual field. We now know, however, that this is an error. Among the countless possibilities that exist at every moment to structure what is seen, the visual system automatically seeks out the best, most orderly one and presents it to us ready-made. We have no choice any more. That is why we are almost unanimously of the opinion that there is no other alternative organization than the one we see, and do not suspect the miracle that occurs in our senses at every moment. Different perceptual organizations can, however, have quite different strengths, and sometimes several organizations of one and the same stimulus distribution are in competition, among which each possesses a different advantage. In such cases the observer has the opportunity to intervene. Depending on where one fixates

Figure 53A
The grid of dots is a restless pattern because all kinds of different suborganizations compete with each other for dominance without final victory.

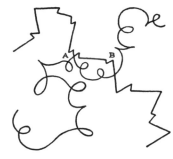

Figure 54
A curly line and a zigzag line? At a first, quick glance, certainly. But if one looks at point A, one thinks, because of the smooth continuation, each line has a zigzagging and a curly half, that only cross accidentally. If one looks away from A to B, then again, as in the first impression, the lines group according to their nature (cf. pages 18 and 23).

in figure 54, it is either the law of good continuation[15] or the law of *good Gestalt,*[16] that is decisive.

1.   CONTRADICTIONS BETWEEN TACTILE AND VISUAL ORGANIZATIONS

The relative strength of different perceptual organizations is not the same for all senses. In one and the same place in the world you might find with your eyes two intersecting circles, but with your fingertips a central core in the form of an almond embedded in a bread roll.[17] This is only because in this case in vision the law of good continuation dominates, whereas in *touch* it is the law of the *common center*[18] that is decisive for the organization. For the same reason one often *feels* in fig-

---

15. See p. 17.
16. See p. 22ff.
17. See p. 16.
18. See p. 22.

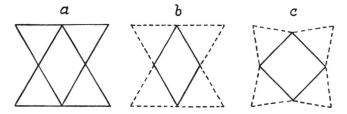

Figure 55

Two intersecting triangles in the adult's visual perception, in which the law of good continuation rules, supplemented by the law of greatest simplicity (a). In touch the same figure structures itself primarily according to the law of the common center into a rectangular core and a serrated wreath; there arises a star (b), which often generates quite a regular impression (c, drawn by 10-year-olds). Younger children even *see* a star here. (From J. Becker: *Über taktil-motorische Figurwahrnehmung. Psychol. Forschg.* 20, 1934.)

ure 55a[19] a star instead of two crossed triangles, that is a rectangle with four spikes around it (figure 55b); some observers may even have the impression that the star is quite regular (figure 55c).

In other cases where visually the law of good continuation determines the percept, with touch, different shapes are perceived because here the law of closure[20] dominates. Thus in seeing there arises in one and the same figure a wavy line and a crenellated line that cross each other several times (figure 56a), whereas in touch you usually perceive a row of approximately rectangular closed cells, that touch each other (figure 56b); or visually, you perceive a zigzag intersected by a straight line that connects its ends (figure 57a), whereas by touch, it is three triangles touching each other that is perceived, and you hardly ever notice that the sides of each pair of triangles joining each other all lie on a straight line (figures 57b and c). For the same reason the curly line (figure 58a) resembles by touch mostly the image of a zigzag stalk with leaves; it has the effect of a serrated or wavy line, on which closed cells sit alternately left and right (figure 58b).

2. Laws of Structure in Children

It is generally true that the law of good continuation is more important in vision than in touch. This is probably related to the idea that the sense

---

19. How the image is produced for touch is described on p. 15.

20. See pp. 10 and 21.

Figures 56–58
Figures that visually (in adults) are structured predominantly according to the law of good continuation, but in touch more likely according to the law of closure.

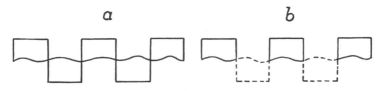

Figure 56
Wavy line and crenellated line (a) perceived in the tactile sense usually as a row of approximately rectangular closed cells (b). (Figure from M. Wertheimer: *Untersuchungen zur Lehre von der Gestalt*, II. *Psychol. Forschg.* 4, 1923.)

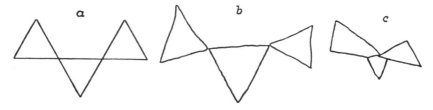

Figure 57
Zigzag crossed by a straight line (a) perceived in the tactile sense predominantly as three closed triangles, usually without straight-line continuations (b, c). (From unpublished experiments of J. Becker.)

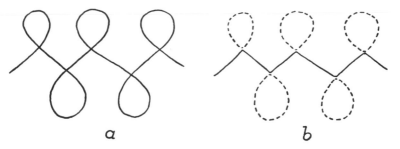

Figure 58
Curly line (a) perceived in the tactile sense as a type of zigzag stalk with leaves: five rings on a zigzagging line (b).

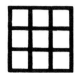

Figure 59

Grid, in the vision of an adult is typically a rectangular frame with two pairs of parallel bars in it that cross each other. The law of good continuation rules unchallenged; other laws such as closure work only as ancillary influences. But compare the following figures from touch experiments with an actual grid that is about twice as large. (Figures 59a, 60, 61 from H. Volkelt: *Neue Untersuchungen über die kindliche Auffassung und Wiedergabe von Formen. Ber. 4. Kongr. Heilpäd.* in Leipzig, 1928, Berlin, 1929.)

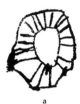
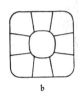
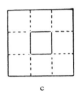

a b c

Fig. 60 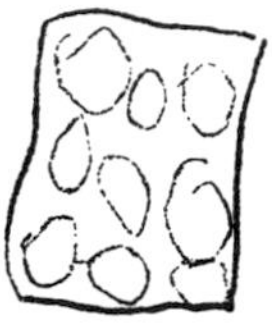 Fig. 61

Figure 60

The same grid as in figure 59, but in a touch experiment with a 6-year-old child, organized according to the law of the common center: two rings with individual connecting lines emerge. (a) The child's drawing after touching the grid in figure 59. (b) Transitional form between the pattern of center-surround organization (c) and the drawing (a), to make clear how the child's drawing may be thought to have arisen. (c) The center-surround organization is drawn veridically into the image of the pattern.

Figure 61

"Frame with lots of holes inside." Correct representation of the grid (figure 59) when the law of closure alone determines its organization. Drawing by a child between 4 and 6 years of age in the touch experiment.

of touch was arrested at a more primitive stage of development than vision. Traces of this development of the senses can be found in the life of the human individual.

If the above-mentioned touch experiments are performed on approximately ten-year-old children, a further decrease occurs in the effect of the law of good continuation; structural organizations of the kinds shown in figures 55b, 56b, and 57b become more frequent. In touch experiments with four- to six-year-olds, those organizations are found almost exclusively. To the extent that these children are able to draw at least partially valid likenesses of figures such as the simple grid of figure 59, the law of the common center (figure 60) or the law of closure (figure 61) determines the structure for them. It would be rash to dismiss a child's drawing like figure 60a as simply wrong. The structure of an outer and an inner ring with a common center, which are tied together by eight single lines (figure 60b), is in principle just as correct as the organization into a frame with 2 × 2 crossed inner bars, as the adult sees it. Aside from the rounding off of the rings, which perhaps also reflects a child's impression quite correctly, the only crude error is that the number of connecting lines comes out too large (compare figure 60b). Also the child who, after feeling the same grid by touch, has drawn (by the child's own description) "many holes" (figure 61) has by no means done anything wrong, but rather has just perceived the pattern as organized strictly according to the law of closure.

With still younger children the law of the common center often determines the figural organization in seeing as well, whereas for adults it is the law of good continuation that is decisive. When an alert three and a half-year-old was given figure 55a, and further circle groups as in figures 62a and 63a, to look at and was asked what it was, the child replied without hesitation, "Those are strange stars." Accordingly, the child saw these figures as organized from the center (figures 62b and 63b). To be sure, when asked again a few minutes later, the circle figures (figures 62a and 63a) were now called "rings" (which in the child's vocabulary meant circles). In spite of the quick change of the percept, it remains significant that the figures could be seen as starlike at all, and that indeed that is the way they looked at first glance.

Why the sense of good continuation at crossings and forks is so much more strongly disrupted, especially at earlier developmental stages of the senses, than in the vision of adults is at this point open to conjecture. The most likely explanation would be that closed-line strokes in perception are usually not figures[21] themselves, but serve only as borders.[22] What one actually sees is the more or less wide and robust flat surface area that those borders excise from the ground and surround. By contrast, open, branching, and many crossing (and all self-crossing) line strokes have the tendency in perception to attain the status of figure. But such figures are never wider than—just a line. Their delicacy and fragility immediately stand out, especially in branching structures.[23] And

21. See p. 6.
22. See p. 7.
23. See figure 30, p. 22.

Figures 62 and 63

Two figures which in the perception of the adult are composed of many circles according to the laws of good continuation and greatest simplicity—but by a 3½-year-old child. As with figure 55, they were described as "strange stars"; that is, they were seen by the child as structured according to the law of the common center into inner and outer parts. (From J. Becker; see figure 55.)

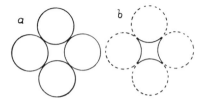

Figure 62
Four circles touching each other (a). With the inner-outer organization in the perception of the child, the same figure is a quadrangle with a curved wreath (b).

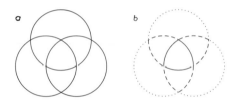

Figure 63
Three circles crossing each other several times (a). With the inner-outer organization in the child's perception, it is a triangle with spikes and a curved wreath (b).

that is probably the reason why structures of this type cannot persist well in less-developed senses.

People often say that children live in a different world, without thinking of anything particular about such a statement. Here we have captured clearly only one of the many differences between the world of children and that of adults. We now know that the same things not only often can make a very different impression* on children, but also that very different things are present in their experience compared with ours. Fortunately it is not always thus, but only where certain laws of vision come into conflict with one another. Wherever they work together in the same direction, we can still count on the borders of objects to behave in the same way for children as they do for us. For objects of particular significance, one's fellow humans, for example, the perceptual segmentation of children and adults will differ only under unfavorable circumstances, such as possibly in disorderly crowds. The laws of organization are the same, of course, for children and adults. It is only their relative weight that is somewhat different.

---

* For example numbers and other such forms that we see as dead and indifferent often look animated for them: sad or happy, proud or humble, etc.

3.   STRUCTURAL RELATIONSHIPS AT THE EDGES OF THE VISUAL FIELD

For our further conclusions we will no longer rely on the testimony of young children, which is often difficult to interpret, but rather proceed in a generally more accessible way. Not only the different senses of a living creature, but even different parts of the same sense organ, are often developed differently. On the whole, our entire body surface is sensitive to touch. But for fine touch we ordinarily use only the tips of the fingers. In order to see something precisely, we must direct our gaze to it. It is not enough that the image falls just anywhere in the eye, but rather it must be brought to the finest and most highly developed locus at the center of the back of the eye, the fovea or retinal pit. Surrounding this spot are areas of gradually decreasing acuity of resolution. This explains our observation in figure 54 that the law of good continuation weakens as soon as the place where the lines come together is no longer near the fixation point.

Farther out, the structure becomes ever weaker and cruder, as occurs also with the sense of touch. The borders become blurred. The unifying effect of proximity[24] becomes overwhelming. The color difference must become ever stronger and the distance to the next color change ever larger, if independent percepts are still to be discernible. Smaller distances and weaker color changes,[25] which in the region of the fixation point determine the intrafigural organization of things, no longer act as borders and segregations, and therefore no longer generate perceived forms.[26] If the distances and color differences are not too small or too weak, however, they cause an imbalance and restlessness in each intrafigural organization that is difficult to describe and can best be compared with what in clearly seen objects is called their grain, or texture, the material nature of their perceived structure. You see in that region an impression of textural properties such as stripes, zigzags, knotted or finely perforated textures, that often contain very specific hints of shapes, but *precisely only hints*, no clearly segregated, countable, or above all, *individually identifiable component parts* such as actual stripes, spikes, knots, holes, and the like.

More generally, it no longer surprises us when we find this kind of relationship in the perception of younger children, even for patterns

24. See pp. 12, 29 section 1.

25. See p. 33, and p. 34, figure 47.

26. See p. 15f.

Figure 64

Representation of the grid (figure 59) in touch experiments with children 5 to 6 years of age who do not really want to reproduce the single elements of the whole, but rather the configuration of its constituent component parts. One child (drawing a) declares approximately "inside it is knotty," which is intended to convey the impression of the crossings (the center ring is supposed to indicate this); "around this there are holes" (the winglike objects); "at the outer edge there are corners" (the small tips). The other child (drawing b) draws almost the same picture as figure 60a (closed and organized around the common center), but adds on the outside a number of lines to indicate explicitly that there are corners there. (From H. Volkelt; see figure 59.)

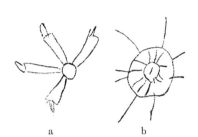
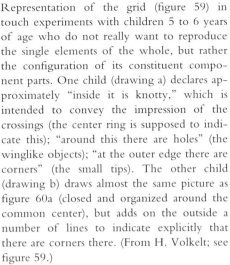

a   b

that appear clearly structured to an adult who looks directly at them. When very young children, under four to six years of age, try to reproduce images such as figure 59, their drawings often reveal that they are not intended to be structurally faithful reproductions, but rather (at least in part) they are attempts to express somehow the properties of the total object that stand intermediate between form and hue (figure 64). It is not only the awkwardness of the hand that prevents these children from reproducing veridically the seen or touched objects. The main impediment is that they see mostly material properties that are spread out over entire areas rather than specifically structured component parts, even in fairly simple line patterns.

It is possible to put yourself approximately in the perceptual position of a child by arranging for a drawing like figure 55 to be slid into the visual field on a uniform background from the periphery without knowing ahead of time which drawing it is, and attempting to draw what you see in peripheral vision *without turning your eyes toward it*. For most people this requires some practice, others never master it at all.[27] Even when it works, it is usually not much better than when someone without artistic

27. See the end of this section. Whoever is not successful in peeking around the corner in the requisite manner will find in section 5 an experiment that leads more effortlessly to the same goal.

training attempts to draw a face and thereby tries to reproduce faithfully the friendliness of that face.

It is no use trying to move the figures progressively outward from the fixation point to observe the point at which certain colors or features abruptly disappear in the periphery. For under these conditions, surprisingly, you often notice certain visual properties way out to the edge of the visual field, whose perception actually could be achieved only within a region near the fixation point. That is also why under natural conditions the world, even at the edge of the visual field, does not look gray like the fading edge of an old vignette photograph, but appears just as vividly colored as it does at the central portion of the visual field, even though it actually should not be permitted to, because the eyes have no or only a few scattered color sensitive-cells in the corresponding regions (figure 65).

4. MOTION AS THE STRONGEST SEGREGATING POWER

Toward the outer boundaries of the visual field the coherence of everything seen becomes so strong that only the strongest segregating powers

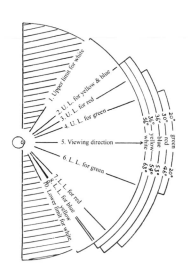

Figure 65

Distribution of spectral sensitivity in a perpendicular cross section through the visual field of a normal eye (after Hoeber: *Lehrbuch der Physiologie*). For measurement, small colored disks are presented on a perimetric arc through the visual field. The arrow → indicates the viewing direction. A yellow-green disk, for example, when the movement begins at the top, would look like a whitish speck in the direction of 1, whereas from 2 on it would appear colored, but first purely yellow; only from 4 onward would it have its correct yellow-green color. The boundaries are slightly different in each eye; the boundaries for yellow and blue do not always coincide. See also notes 17 and 18. The small print in figure 65 reads as follows: 1. Upper limit for white, 2. U.l. for blue and yellow, 3. U.l. for red, 4. U.l. for green, 5. Direction of gaze, 6. Lower limit for green, 7. L.l. for red, 8. 9. L.l. for blue and yellow. 10. L.l. for white; eye; green, red, blue, yellow, white.

can make something emerge as an independent object from the surround. With images of moderate size even the most prominent color contrast that (except for light sources) occurs at objects in our environment is finally no longer sufficient. Smaller and fainter objects disappear closer to the fovea, whereas larger objects with stronger contrast vanish near the periphery, and only visual motion against the background can make them visible again.[28] That which is immobile in its surround disappears from view, and only with renewed movement will it reappear.

This characteristic of our perception has a very significant consequence; namely, that, except from nearby and almost exactly in the direction of the gaze, one either does not see the turn signals on automobiles at all, or cannot distinguish them from side mirrors and the like,[29] if one does not happen to glance at them the moment they are turned up. [Translators' note: Automobile turn signals of the era were not blinking lights, but were like small paddles that swung up into view and remained static.] But it would be easy to remedy this. If, instead of remaining immobile after being turned up, turn indicators remained in constant motion, they would be visible from a much greater distance and in peripheral vision, even for the slightly nearsighted and the colorblind. It would then be possible in one glance to see everything of significance in heavy and fast traffic at busy intersections where it is hard to get an overview, and thereby avoid nasty surprises. In some vehicles (for example, Berlin buses) for years turn indicators were attached in such a way that the jerk of turning them up kept them oscillating up and down for a while afterward. This kind of indicator should be made generally mandatory.

The described role of movement has long been known in the sense of touch. During gentle movements you do not notice your clothes soon after getting dressed unless they do not fit properly. That this phenomenon is not just a matter of simple ignoring, can be demonstrated by a simple experiment. If you wrap a fairly loose rubber band around the middle of your lower arm, you first feel the pressure sharply delineated and distributed clearly in the form of a ring. But it soon loses its shape and sharpness and becomes a hazy "pressure cloud." After a while, even with focused attention, there is nothing left to notice. But as soon as the ring is displaced even slightly, its shape immediately flashes back with its original sharpness. Of course, one must do this experiment with eyes closed, and have the band moved by another person.

---

28. Law of common fate, p. 35.

29. And this occurs, as figure 65 shows, despite the striking red color.

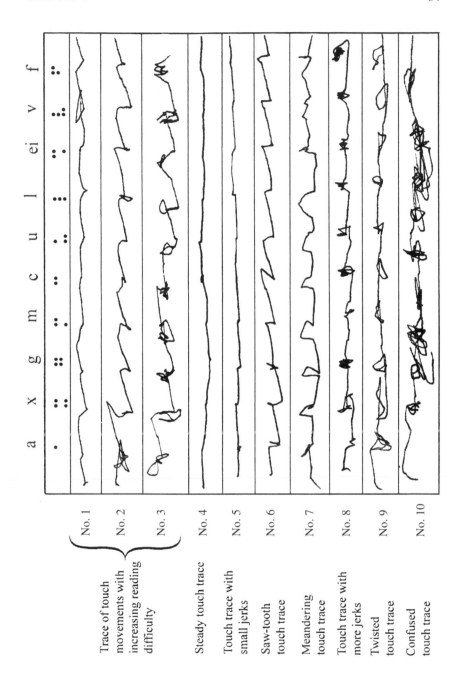

It speaks anew for the lower level of development of the sense of touch that these relationships prevail even in the most sophisticated tactile task. The blind person who reads Braille with the fingertips always does so with gentle rubbing motions. If you force him to place the fingers on the Braille without motion, he recognizes nothing, or only with effort the simplest forms (e.g., a single dot or dash). For a long time it was thought that with these reading motions, the blind person traces from one dot to another, connects and counts the dots in his mind, and recognizes their relative positions from the direction of his own movements. But on closer study, it turned out that it is sometimes possible to identify the reader from the characteristic pattern of hand motions (and, of course, one can judge the clarity of the Braille from those motions), but not—as might be expected—what letters are being read (figure 66). The real purpose of the sliding motions of the fingers is to displace the entire tactile stimulus across the pressure-sensitive surface of the fingers, because only with continuous movement do the raised parts of the touched surface remain sharply segregated enough and thus clearly structured. You can easily demonstrate this to yourself with homemade groups of Braille dots.[30]

It would be a mistake to think that in the above experiments the only thing that is perceived is motion, from which the presence of certain shapes is inferred. Rather, motion has under certain circumstances the astonishing power to segregate things from their surroundings so sharply that their shape becomes immediately evident. Under unfavorable conditions of course—such as in the appearance or disappearance of an object when the movement is over too quickly, or in vision when it occurs too far out toward the periphery of the visual field—you still see only that at a certain place something is happening. This literally means that something did indeed become segregated from its surround,

---

30. Figure 66 contains examples of Braille signs; for how you can produce them yourself, see p. 15.

◄ **Figure 66**

Finger movements during reading of Braille; about $\frac{2}{3}$ actual size. On top are the signs (a, x, g, m, c, u, l, ei, v, f). Below are the movements of the right index finger while reading these symbols. The weaker the reader (and the less clear the writing), the longer the reader has to go back and forth across the symbol; for the best reader a single glide over it suffices. There is no correlation at all between the shape of the symbol and the shape of the corresponding reading movement. (From K. Bürklen: *Das Tastlesen der Blindenpunktschrift. Z. Ang. Psychol. Beih.* 16, 1917.)

but without yet assuming sharp borders and thus a clear form. The most prominent characteristic of what is happening is the irresistible urge with which our gaze is drawn to it, as long as we remain ignorant of its nature. Not shape and color, but rather such forces that entice and urge certain specific behavior are perhaps the earliest characteristics of all perception. Hence this reveals its close relationship with the most primitive sensory performance of all, the so-called reflex, which in the purest case is completely devoid of perception, and which in response to specific sensory stimulation triggers the corresponding bodily activity in the absence of conscious volition. There is a continuous gradation between conscious behavior and unconscious reflexes.

5. THE SEGREGATION OF SMALLEST AND FAINTEST IMAGES

It should be clear by now that you cannot present lines in the visual field and say that up to one point one law of perception rules, from another point a different one dominates, beyond a third point movement is necessary for the perception of Gestalten, and beyond a final point no forms are perceived at all any more. The larger an object is, and the stronger its contrast against the background, the longer it will survive as a perceived form as it drifts into peripheral vision.[31] And vice versa, for ever smaller objects with ever lower contrast, the boundaries of perceivability move ever closer in toward the fixation point. Eventually at the smallest perceivable size or contrast, the experience assumes ever more primitive forms *even in the region of the fixation point itself.*[32] The relationships that prevail here have been only partly explored, but this much is already certain.

If you try to describe or draw the interior of greatly reduced figures that you have never seen before full size, the result is much like in the description (see section 3) of figures seen in peripheral vision (figures 67–70). The interior is unstructured, but characterized by properties such as "confusion, lattice-like, jelly-like" (Sander). Characteristics that have their very definite place in the full-size and full-contrast figure are

---

31. This holds true also for boundaries of color sensitivity. The numbers in figure 65 are valid precisely only for small colored disks that are used in the perimeter for investigating the visual field.

32. This is also true for the perception of colors; tiny color spots that are not too bright are seen at the fixation point of a trichromatic eye only as bright, no longer colored.

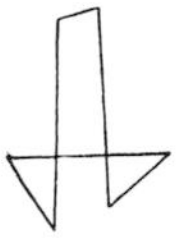

Figure 67

A stimulus pattern used to test the perception of the smallest Gestalten. (Figures 67–70 from E. Wohlfahrt: *Der Auffassungsvorgang an kleinen Gestalten. N. Psychol. Stud.* 4, 1932.)

Figures 68–70

Attempts of three observers to portray how figure 67 looks with maximum reduction in size; of course, the observers had not seen the figure full size before. As in figure 64, these drawings are not to be taken literally, because they too represent only attempts to express in a drawing the properties that appear to extend out over the whole, or over certain parts of it.

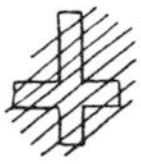

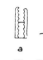

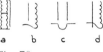

Fig. 68 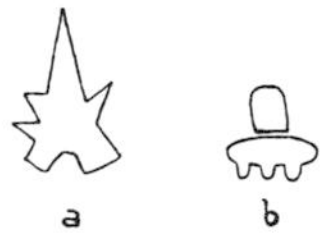   Fig. 69   Fig. 70

Figure 68

The observer sees something crosslike, but it is related as a whole to a striving toward the upper right. The diagonal lines are intended to represent this.

Figure 69

(a) Another observer first sees something ascending, spiked, a type of star whose upward-oriented point is longer; the jaggedness can of course be represented in the drawing only by many single spikes. (b) With a somewhat weaker reduction the figure becomes structured into two distinct parts: an upright beam above and a horizontal part below; however, at the lower part, a diffusely spread jaggedness still prevails.

Figure 70

For a third observer, diffusely extended texture and genuine segregation alternate in particular regions of the figure. (a) First he sees two vertical beams that are connected somewhere in the middle or below. But at the same time the entire figure is jagged. In a telling manner the spikes spreading out over the figure are drawn inside the figure. (b) Suddenly the left side becomes genuinely structured: the vertical is straight, and lower down, after a break, there is a true spike to the left. On the right, by contrast, the spatially extended jaggedness initially persists. (c) The extended jaggedness disappears even on the right, but the lower part still retains a true spike there. (d) With prolonged viewing the spike point again becomes unclear, disappears and the jaggedness is once again spread out, blurred. It even remains this way as a new description is given—the left beam appears to pierce through the curve.

often spread out in a blurred way over the whole, or over subparts of the whole, in the reduced stimulus, "without regard to the number and the structural relation to each other of their bearers" (Wohlfahrt). Such experiments are most easily performed with a reversed telescope.

Even in the direction of gaze we see very small (and also very distant) objects only *if they are moving*. We are not better here than the frog, which lets the most alluring fly sit undisturbed in front of its nose as long as it does not move. Any hunter or soldier can testify to that. Whoever freezes and stays motionless in open country when they hear suspicious noises, and whoever waves at departing friends at the train station, makes use of this experience. You can test yourself without going into the countryside, hunting, or to the train station. Just make a couple of fine dots on a piece of writing paper, then lay a sheet of translucent paper over it: the dots disappear. If you now move the covering sheet back and forth a bit, the dots are suddenly visible again if they are sufficiently prominent. If you look at a fiber of the moving translucent sheet, the covered dots remain just as visible as when you look at them directly. This proves that what you see depends on Gestalt relationships—on commonality and difference in fate—and not on detailed happenings on the retina of the eye. The experiment succeeds quite well if you lay a piece of middleweight typing paper over figure 53 (p. 40), although not the same for all the dots, because of their different contrasts. Anyone experienced in tracing drawings discovers this procedure for making invisible dots visible again.

Even spots of larger extent, which are invisible because of their low contrast at rest, become visible again when they move.[33] But they must be displaced *relative to their background* by the law of common fate. If the background moves with the spot, it remains invisible; if the background moves by itself while the spot itself remains at rest, the spot becomes visible again. And now for the most astonishing experiment.[34] If you lay a tautly stretched piece of tulle over a surface that looks uniform, such as a sheet of photographic paper, and move it back and forth, you can see spots on the covered paper that are not visible when it is not covered.

---

33. The differential threshold with motion, circumstances permitting, amounts to less than half, in experiments by Basler—0.72% of the surround luminance instead of 1.62% at rest.

34. A. Basler: *Über die Verbesserung der Wahrnehmbarkeit wenig unterscheidbarer Flächen auf gleichmäßigem Grunde. Z. Sinnesphysiol.* 66, 1935.

6. A FUNDAMENTAL CONCLUSION

Our overview of the developmental stages of vision, and of the perception of objects altogether, leads to an important general conclusion. The initial task of our senses in the perception of objects is not to combine an assembly of tiny individual sensations into more extensive wholes, as was taught for centuries even to the present by philosophers and psychologists, but rather to break up the initial unity of the sensory field, to subdivide it with boundaries, and to segregate out formed substructures from within it. The individual sensations of that doctrine *never existed in the world*, least of all in the earlier more primitive stages of perception. They are pure thought constructs that are arrived at by taking the natural segregation of the perceptual field achieved by our vision to its extreme limit, regardless of the Gestalt laws. But this exercise of disassembling experience into its component pieces does nothing to advance our understanding of the actual processes in perception, it only makes the problem more difficult.

Even a living body is not composed of a heap of individual cells or limbs, but rather an immense diversity of organs, suborgans, and cells that emerge spontaneously from a single fertilized ovum through continuous furrowing and division. So too in perception; the percept arises not through association, that is, through joining or coupling or, what is exactly the same, through synthesis—the conjoining of simplest parts. This monumental error, which for a long time led science on a fruitless search for "mental elements" (sensations), was not due to improper application of the procedures of natural science to a nonnatural science area, but rather the reverse. The error originates at the philosopher's desk, and it was only by the natural science procedure of the controlled experiment that its weakness came to light. The source of this error can be traced to the way that humans tend to construct things, with wire and string, with nails and screws, with mortar, glue, and paste, assembling whole structures out of elemental parts. It is no wonder therefore that a similar error was committed in the purely humanistic realm where until recently that error was just as common as in psychology: as if one were to believe that the *Iliad* or the *Nibelungenlied* had been created by a collector or organizer stitching together songs that previously existed in isolation into the whole that we know, and no one came to the idea that the whole, in all its abundance, could have unfolded itself out of one unitary core thought.[35]

---

35. Andreas Heusler: *Nibelungensage and Nibelungenlied*, 1. *Aufl.*, Berlin, 1921.

5

GESTALT LAWS SERVING CAMOUFLAGE

1. INVISIBLE ANIMALS

As every hunter knows, you can often search in vain for hours in a familiar place for a familiar animal. If you see it at all, it seems suddenly to pop into existence as if by magic, in a place where a moment ago nothing at all was to be seen of an animal. You often do not trust your own eyes. For the animal that suddenly appeared was not hidden behind grass and foliage such that you could have discovered it only by a lucky chance of seeing an exposed portion of it.[36] Rather, it was sitting there the whole time, life-size and in plain view, and you had surely looked right at it a dozen times without realizing it (figure 71). If it had been a person sitting in the same spot, you would hardly have had to search at all. From far away the person would have immediately caught your eye.

It is obvious that this is related to the colors and patterns of the animal's hide, and sometimes also to its Gestalt. People have long debated whether the primary purpose of markings on some animals is to make them as nearly invisible as possible, or whether the real reason for their appearance is quite different, and only by chance does it also have this effect. Without becoming embroiled in that debate, it is clear that you do not see the bird in figure 71, and we ask how this happens.

2. INCONSPICUOUSNESS IS POOR SEGREGATION: CAMOUFLAGE ACCORDING TO THE LAW OF SIMILARITY

To be inconspicuous, one dresses oneself in inconspicuous colors; thus perhaps certainly not in fiery red, but rather in gray and brownish tones, like a mouse or animals in the forest. Everyone is inclined to view

---

36. Some animals understand with surprising facility how to make themselves invisible by concealing and disguising themselves, and their bodies are covered with special barbs with which they attach themselves to their protective cover (figures 71A and B). They thereby follow most precisely the law of similarity (section 2).

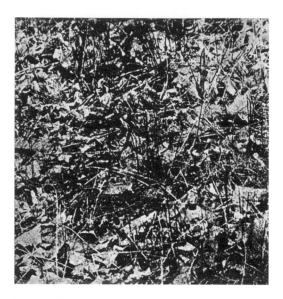

Figure 71

A well-camouflaged animal. The American woodcock (*Philohela minor*) in its nest. If you have the time, first look for it without help, with a stopwatch in your hand; how long did it take? The bird's eye is exactly 2.5 cm from the top and 2.0 cm from the right border of the picture, the bright beak is pointed down toward the right. Basic rule of camouflage: color and fine patterning are similar to the appearance of the dry foliage of the surround, so that the outline is obliterated (see p. 33f, figure 46). The fact that solitary dark stalks cross the image of the bird is not essential; compare figure 37, pp. 25. (From Thayer; see footnote 51.)

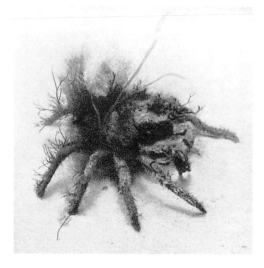

Figure 71A

Camouflage by disguising with foreign material. A sea spider, which for some time has been living in a tank with red algae, has adorned itself all over with lots of red algae. However, the disguise does not work here, since for the purpose of the photograph the animal was taken out of the algae tank and placed on white dune sand. (A, B, C from H. Nitschke: *Wie Tiere sich tarnen. Natur und Volk* 62, 1932.)

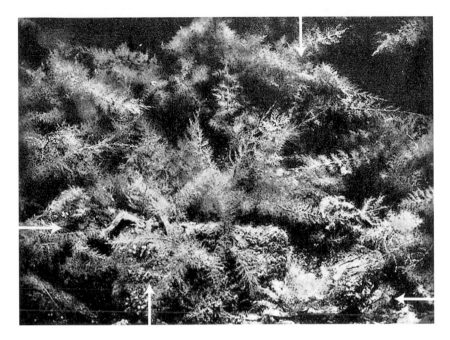

Figure 71B
Two camouflaged sea spiders in appropriate surroundings (at the intersections of the
two pairs of arrows). They did not choose the hydroid polyps for camouflage because they happened to be available, but for reasons of similarity. If one puts these
animals in a tank with algae, they tear off the polyps and replace them with algae. In
a tank with a red bottom that contains brightly colored scraps of paper, they seek
out the red ones and ignore all other colors.

conspicuousness and inconspicuousness as definitive characteristics of
certain colors. But this opinion is wrong. Those characteristics are conspicuous that lead to segregation into figure or object[37] according to
Gestalt laws, which also means that they lead to the formation of correct, appropriate borders[38] in the percept. In the Russian snow a gray
field coat was not the most inconspicuous piece of clothing; what was,
was a long white nightshirt, like the white coat of the polar bear or
snow hare. Whoever wants to hide in a blooming poppy field will find
the brilliant scarlet pantaloons of the former French army uniform just
the right thing. According to the law of similarity,[39] the same color

37. See p. 4.
38. See p. 16.
39. See pp. 32, 38f.

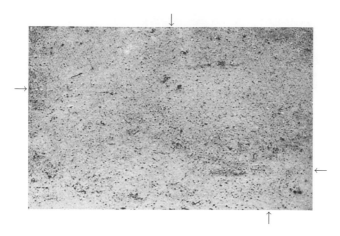

Figure 71C

Turbot in the sand. The two arrows above left show the mouth cleft, the two below right the end of the tail. The fish is not covered with sand, rather it is lying exposed in the open, but it has so taken on the color of the sand that its outline disappears. On a black background it becomes black, on speckled gravel it even becomes speckled, and all this in a time of at most two hours.

without a border merges into its environment.[40] This is the reason why no color is intrinsically inconspicuous; each color is inconspicuous only in the correct environment. That is why snow animals are white, grass animals green, and desert animals yellowish and brown. And this is not just in general and approximately. In studies of caterpillars, for example, one is repeatedly surprised how the color of their host plant—of its leaves, blossoms, stems, or fruit, each according to its way of life, is mirrored to the finest nuances in the caterpillar's markings.[41]

The best protective coloring is of course a changeable one, as seen in several flat fish (cf. figure 71C) and many small shrimp that after some time take on the coloring (and to some extent even the pattern) of the ground in which they happen to find themselves. How these animals manage to do this is an extremely difficult and complicated matter. At any rate it is now known with certainty that it is not simply the environment somehow being mirrored in the animal's skin, but that vision plays a role. Blinded animals no longer match their color to their environment.

If an object is to be hidden by blurring its boundaries, then it is important that besides the coloring, its texture and fine detail are

---

40. See figure 71C.

41. Compare especially K. Dietze (cited with figure 74).

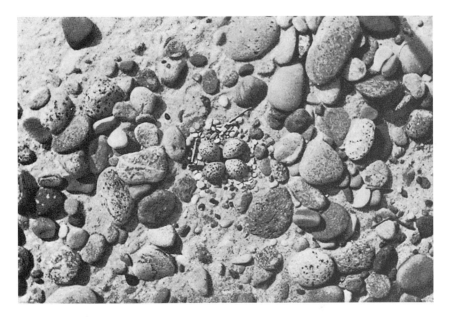

Figure 71D
The eggs of a ringed plover are well camouflaged, although their outlines are perfectly sharp and not blurred. According to the law of belongingness they are firmly integrated into the sea of stones on the beach. The searching eye sees only a few more stones (cf. part 3, p. 67). (From O. and A. Koehler: *Brütende Sandregenpfeifer. Natur und Volk* 65, 1935.)

matched to those of its environment. Who would have thought that it is precisely by *covering*—at least from the bird's perspective—that one could make oneself especially visible? Every soldier learns that he must not simply pull the tent cover smoothly over his foxhole, but should throw it over it so as to be as rumpled and folded as possible. Because by the law of similarity, a smooth area segregates itself from a rumpled environment just as effectively as a yellow region segregates from a blue one. It is beneficial when a bird that is brooding in dry leaves has the color of the dry leaves, but even better when it is spotted like a pile of dry leaves (figure 71). The butterfly that rests on old tree trunks does not just have the dull brown color of the bark, but often also mimics in great detail the characteristic spots, cracks, peeled-off areas, and small lichens (figure 72) of the texture of the bark. Some animals are so incredibly well camouflaged by suppression of their boundaries due to their similar color and fine texture that you would think it must be their life's purpose to play at being hidden (figure 73). To be sure, a further basic

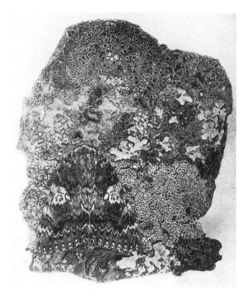

Figure 72
The dark crimson underwing butterfly (*Catocala sponsa* L.) is also camouflaged according to the law of similarity. Coloring and fine patterning of this butterfly match so well with the surrounding bark that its outline disappears. Note the mimicking of the small bark lichens on its wings. (From the Senckenberg Museum, Frankfurt am Main.)

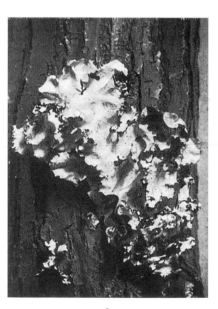

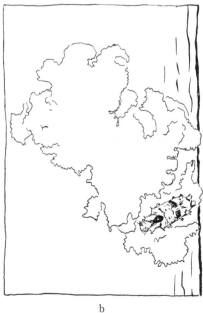

a   b

Figure 73
(a) Where is the beetle sitting? An example of complete camouflage according to the law of similarity: the lichen beetle (*Lithimus nigrocristatus*) from Madagascar. (From the Senckenberg Museum, Frankfurt am Main.) (b) This is how the beetle is sitting on the lichen in figure 73a.

principle of camouflage collaborates more or less strongly here, the principle of tearing up or partitioning, which we will examine more fully later (see section 5).

3. CAMOUFLAGE ACCORDING TO THE LAW OF BELONGINGNESS

You can also make an object disappear from view whose borders are clearly and sharply visible. For this purpose it only needs to seem to belong as a part or element to a larger structure in its surroundings, like the rubber band on the geometric drawing and the pencil on the black mourning border in figure 35. The eggs of the ringed plover (figure 71D), gulls, and sea swallows can under certain circumstances be sharply segregated from the fine gravel on which they lie, but for the searching eye they are just a few more among the thousands of round pebbles on the beach, of which scarcely two are colored and spotted the same. One can hardly assert that the contours of the smooth looper (figure 74a) are obliterated; but the creature sits so stiff and slanting on its stalk as if it were a part of the plant, a narrow leaflet. One must be a botanist and remember that the actual leaves of this plant are shaped quite differently to suspect something is awry. If the butterfly in figure 75 folds its wings together, their borders are indeed less clear than before, but not invisible. Nevertheless you cannot see it any more without effort, for the underside of its wings is marked precisely so that for a naïve observer it seems that there are only a few more leaves on the blooming shrub. In some animals camouflage according to the law of *belongingness* has also advanced to the point that not only their color and patterning, but even their entire body structure follows the pattern, and all the other concerns of a living organism appear to have retreated behind the vital concern of camouflage (figures 76–78).

4. PLAYING DEAD: CAMOUFLAGE ACCORDING TO THE LAW OF COMMON FATE

Countless animals eat only live things. Something that resembles a corpse does not appeal to these animals and is thus ignored. That is what first comes to mind when you watch how a beetle under threat plays dead. However, its motionlessness has yet another much more reliable effect, the entire consequence of which is noticed only by closer research into the laws of vision: playing dead is a means of camouflage, and one of

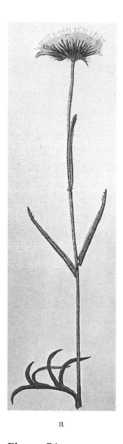
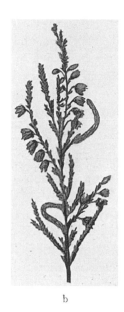

a   b

Figure 74
(a) The three leaves in the middle of the scabious stem are three caterpillars (*Eupithecia scabiosata* BKH. of the Bergstrasse). (b) This heather also has a small branch at the top right that is not authentic, but that on closer examination resolves itself into a looper (*Eupithecia narata* gen. aest. from the Zurich region). Despite sharply visible outlines it is well camouflaged according to the law of belongingness (figures 28, 33–35, p. 20ff). Only the botanist who knows that the leaves of the scabious are shaped differently and furthermore are not located in the middle of the flower stem notices that something is not right. (From K. Dietze: *Biologie der Eupithecien*. 1. T., Berlin, 1910.)

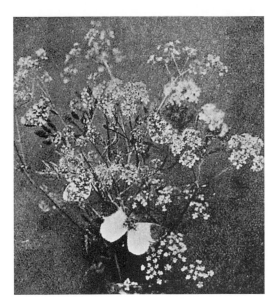

Figure 75
Even the orange-tip butterfly (*Euchloe cardamines*) with folded wings camouflages itself according to the law of belongingness. If you look at the right border of the
picture or look at it from 2 meters distance, all you see, aside from the unfolded butterfly at the bottom, are more umbels of the fool's parsley. (From Thayer; see footnote 51.)

the most effective at that.[42] The beetle that plays dead becomes completely invisible for most observers. For many animals without a highly
developed visual sense, it is invisible under all circumstances (many of
these creatures might perhaps even eat dead animals if only they could
see them), and for creatures with highly developed vision, the motionless
beetle remains invisible at least from a greater distance, or when their
gaze is not by chance directed exactly toward the potential victim or its
immediate neighborhood.

That one is inconspicuous when one remains as nearly motionless
as possible is also understood intuitively by the human. But even that is
only partially correct. Just as no color is intrinsically inconspicuous, so
too no behavior is intrinsically inconspicuous under all circumstances.
One cannot simply assert that motion by its very nature is more conspicuous than rest. When everything is in motion, then according to the law

---

42. See p. 52 section 4, and p. 58.

Figures 76–78
The entire body structure in the service of camouflage according to the law of belongingness.

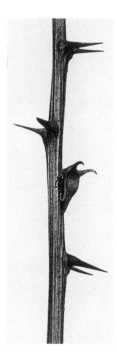

Figure 76
The Brazilian tree hopper (*Hemiptera punctata*) on an acacia twig with double thorns is itself a double thorn. Only someone who is familiar with the regular arrangement of the real thorns notices that there is one too many. (From the Senckenberg Museum, Frankfurt am Main.) The pictured creature is sitting on the twig of a German acacia and even there is not badly camouflaged. Probably the thorns of the Brazilian host plant are much more similar to the creature: slightly bent and broad-bottomed.

of *common fate*[43] anything that remains motionless segregates itself most prominently as a unit from its environment and thus becomes "conspicuous." And for animals with simpler vision, it becomes visible in the first place. It is by this principle that a mind reader finds the man who is hiding some secret, because to his trained eye that man is the only one in the crowd of excited people who, in an effort to be inconspicuous, behaves especially passively. The wisdom that is lacking in the behavior of this man—and indeed of anyone in a similar situation—is evident in the behavior of many animals. For example, the great bittern and several kinds of herons, when they do not stand still in the midst of the swaying reed thicket, but bob untiringly from one leg to the other in synchrony with the surrounding stalks. For with exactly this movement they become invisible in their moving environment. Here it becomes clear

43. See p. 35.

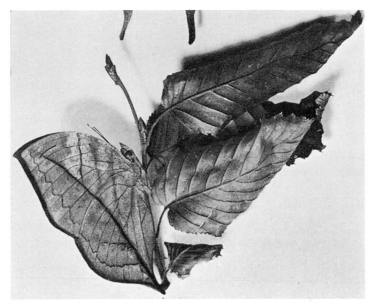

Figure 77
The pair of wings of the Indian leaf butterfly *Kallima paralecta*, which has a preference for living among dry leaves. Seen from below, it has been completely transformed into a withered leaf with stalk, middle rib, and side ribs. (From the Senckenberg Museum, Frankfurt am Main.)

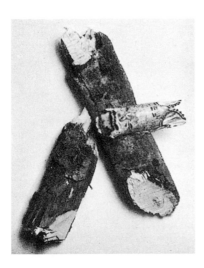

Figure 78
Another masterpiece of camouflage according to the law of belongingness. One of the twigs with both ends broken off is a butterfly with folded wings (the buff-tip or tip moth, *Phalera bucephala*). The end of the head and moon spots on the wing tips mimic the splintered ends of a twig. (From the Senckenberg Museum, Frankfurt am Main.)

again that inconspicuous is that which does not stand out in its environment, because according to its nature (in the most general sense) it belongs to that environment.

It is nearly impossible to take natural pictures of camouflage due to the law of common fate that really shows what is possible in this area. For when the camouflage is complete, you do not see the animal until it flees, and then it is too late for a photo. And if it had been possible to photograph it earlier, the camouflage was not perfect. The Senckenberg Museum in Frankfurt am Main has a photo of a bittern that has been placed strangely tilted next to a pair of equally tilted stalks. This pose is intended to show how the living bird mimics the swaying of the reeds (figure 79).

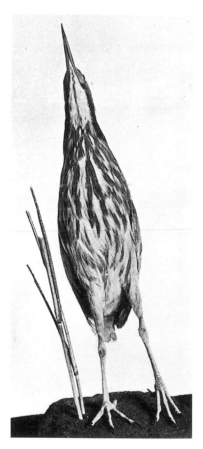

Figure 79
Camouflage according to the law of common fate. The American bittern (*Botaurus lentiginosus* MONT.) in reeds. In spite of the vertical stripes that so nicely mirror the appearance of the reed bank (compare section 6, figures 92–94), the bird would stand out in moving reeds because of its stillness. So it moves with the reeds and thus under natural conditions becomes invisible because of this movement. (Diorama in the Senckenberg Museum, Frankfurt am Main.)

5. The Purpose of Dappling: Camouflage through
Partitioning

Most of the previous examples could, somewhat imprecisely, be explained in the old sense of inconspicuousness. But what about coarsely
dappled animals, black and white cows, auks, and penguins? What about
the white cotton tail of the field hare? One can scarcely imagine more
conspicuous patterns. Could such patterns be protective colorings? Does
their existence not prove that there really are animals that make do without the advantages of inconspicuous coloring, even though many of
them need it as much as their more fortunate relatives?

One Shrove Tuesday I looked out of the window toward the
street at twilight and could not believe my eyes, for hanging obliquely
across the street was a clothes line hung with white laundry, which
under closer observation suddenly changed itself into a tired white horse
standing there, hitched to a vegetable wagon (figure 80). What previously had looked like the gaps between pieces of white laundry were
the bridle and blanket that, somewhat crumpled together, were hanging
over the horse's back. Granted, if a hungry wolf had been standing in
my position that did not know that one does not generally hang laundry
in the street even on Shrove Tuesday, it would have, since it had no use
for laundry, searched further and would despite its hunger have left the
horse alone.[44] The illusion occurred because the dark parts of the harness
happened to be of the same brightness as the street, and thus according
to the law of similarity, the street and the harness merged and became
background, so that only the bright sections of the hide remained as
actual things,[45] indeed as segregated single objects.

In the same way, the colors of jungle birds that in our drab environment are so conspicuous make their wearers invisible in the colored
shimmering lights of southern forests. Certain parts of their bodies,
which match the colors of the surrounding environment, thereby become visually cut out of the body and assigned to the background, so
that the visible remainder takes on an irregular shape not characteristic
of an animal. Strictly speaking, the orange-tip butterfly (figure 75) is
an example. For what is an umbel other than a collection of small,

---

44. As in all further examples, it is of course assumed that hearing and especially
smell are not at work. For predators with a sharp sense of smell and hearing, what
has been said holds only with a quiet stance and favorable wind direction.

45. See p. 2.

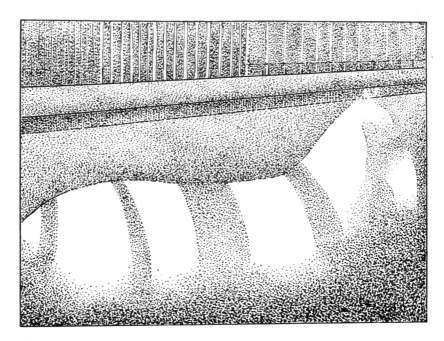

Figure 80
Camouflage effect of dappling: tearing up of the image into irrelevant pieces. Instead of the white horse one sees in the twilight at first glance a clothes-line hung with white laundry. The dark parts of the harness blur into the dark ground and join up to become part of the background; the visible parts of the bright hide remain as disconnected single figures.

bright, little figures through which one can see the background (which seen from above is mostly dark)? We have discussed the butterfly, for in it the visible remainders fit in to conform to their environment quite inconspicuously as an umbel according to the law of belongingness.

By the same principle as that used by dappled animals, heavy artillery is camouflaged in the open by painting it with large conspicuous blobs. This strategy was introduced during the war [WWI] to the greatest astonishment of the uninitiated, and the artillery was better hidden than had it been painted with the most inconspicuous shade of gray.[46]

Breaking up the outline with large spots can be even more thorough. Try, for example, *without reading further*, to figure out what is presented in figures 81–83. Perhaps you see brush with dry branches (figure

46. The camouflaging effect of segregation was discovered around 1900 by G. and A. Thayer (see footnote 51); but their work became known here only later.

Figures 81–83
Puzzling images with which the fox is confronted in nature when it goes hunting at twilight. This is how the pieces of various landscapes in figures 84–86 would look when visibility is poor, e.g. in peripheral vision, or when it is somewhat dark or foggy.

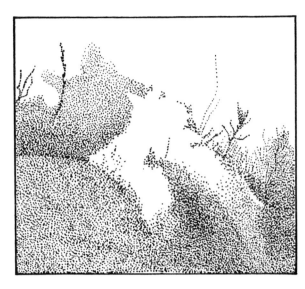

Figure 81
What is this? Undergrowth with dry twigs?

No, a field hare seen from behind, the same as in figures 84 and 87.

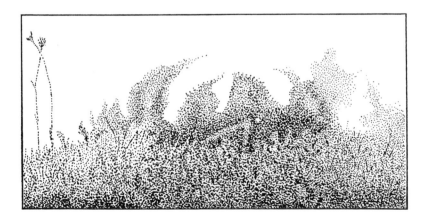

Figure 82
What is this? Large-leafed weeds?

No, a common skunk, the same as in figures 85 and 88.

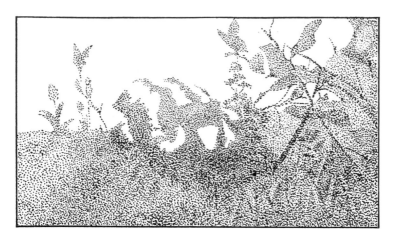

Figure 83
What is this? Young shrubs and bushes?

Yes, but in between is a striped skunk, the same as in figures 86 and 89.

81), some kind of large-leafed weeds (figure 82), loose bushes of umbels and young shrubs (figure 83). In figures 84–86 somewhat better perceptual conditions prevail (with the same direction of gaze and lighting). Nonetheless, you can scarcely see at first glance that a rabbit (seen from behind) and a common or striped skunk are before your eyes. These are all conspicuously colored animals. At the location where a white-dappled animal sits, white spots stand out from the environment, at least to a human who looks from above. These spots attract attention, even if they are not characteristic of the shape of an animal (figures 87–89). But if you see the same animal from ground level at twilight in an open area—as animal enemies most often view each other—under favorable conditions the suspicious bright remaining spots have disappeared. Then it is not only the dark parts of the pattern that become effectively part of the dark growth background, as in the white horse. With proper illumination the white spots also join with the adjacent regions of the background by the law of similarity: the bright spots act like parts of the sky. For the observer now nothing suspicious is left, nothing that could remotely remind one of the presence of an animal, only sky and earth, the border of which passes right through the animal. All of these effects reach their maximum effectiveness under poor viewing conditions, from a great distance, or if the gaze is not directed exactly at the animal;[47] and

47. See p. 50 section 3.

Figures 84–86
Segmentation through dappling. Three conspicuously colored animals are shown, the same as in figures 87–89, but from the viewpoint of a stalking fox. The white spots of the pelt merge with their environment, the pale evening sky, and are thus inconspicuous. The animal is completely divided up for the eye; the boundary between sky and earth goes right through the middle of the animal's body. (From Thayer; see footnote 51.)

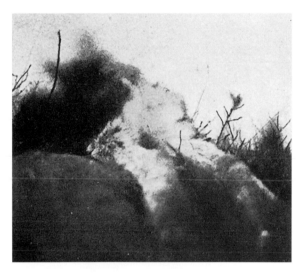

Figure 84
The hare (figure 87) from the fox's point of view. From such a distance you can still see it, but very much worse than if it did not have a white rump. (Dead animal in natural surrounding.)

one surely does not realize how small the area of the highest acuity is in the eye[48] (figures 81–83). The white tail of the rabbit, one of the most conspicuous spots from the direction of view of a human observer, is thus an especially important part of its camouflage against its animal enemies.

Just as you might expect, therefore, animals with dappled hides are especially numerous in regions that exhibit glaring contrasts between light and dark: at the edge of snow fields, at rocky coasts of polar regions, in rocky debris of high mountains and the beach. The ptarmigan (figure 90) with its irregularly spotted transitional plumage disinte-

---

48. In humans, its width is about $2°$ and its height about $1\frac{1}{2}°$.

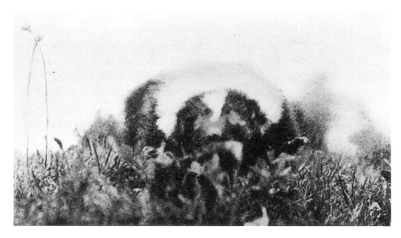

Figure 85
The common skunk (figure 88) from the fox's point of view. If you do not look carefully, all you see is a pair of earth humps and you do not notice that an animal is sitting there. (Stuffed animal outdoors.)

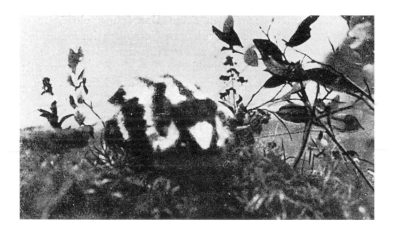

Figure 86
The striped skunk, which in figure 89 would not be overlooked by humans, has as good as disappeared from the fox's view; it is completely divided up into sky and earth by plant growth. (Stuffed animal outdoors.)

Figures 87–89
White dappled animals in a dark environment, from the usual viewpoint of a human observer. The camouflage is poor or entirely lacking. (From Thayer; see footnote 51.)

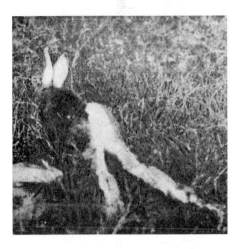

Figure 87
Hare in the grass from behind. The rump merges with the environment (like the horse's harness in figure 80), but the white rear and the ears betray their bearer. (Dead animal in natural setting.)

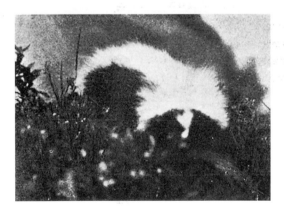

Figure 88
Common skunk on a dark background. Here the white remaining spots hardly look like parts of an animal any more; but they tempt one to look closer and then one can hardly avoid involuntary detection. (Stuffed animal outdoors.)

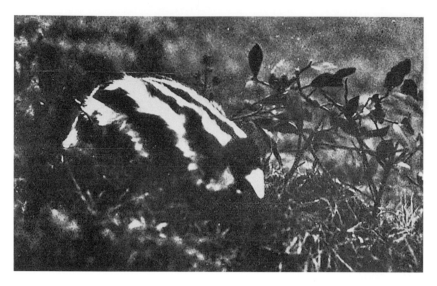

Figure 89
Striped skunk. Here the merging into the dark background occurs only on the lower side. The white stripes on the back actually set off the outline of the animal: the opposite of camouflage is achieved. (Stuffed animal outdoors.)

grates before the observer's eye into patches of damp earth and leftover snow patches. The bright parts of the ringed plover (figure 91) merge seamlessly with the almost equally bright dune sand, and if the nearest stones are similar and close enough, the outer contours of their dark remaining parts also disappear.[49]

6. OTHER LAWS OF VISION USED IN CAMOUFLAGE

1. SUPPRESSION OF WEAK COLOR DIFFERENCES BY NEIGHBORING STRONGER ONES[50]   The bold brightness contrasts in the coats of many dappled animals have yet another important effect. It is not likely, for example, that the white color of the skunk will always match the brightness of the evening sky as precisely as in figure 85. But consider figure

---

49. Even when dark parts of the contour remain, because the nearest stones are too far away or too differently colored, the animal is still camouflaged according to the law of belongingness. The color borders on its plumage run in such a way that the image of the animal disintegrates into individual patches that are rather roundish, resembling pebbles, and therefore become part of them.

50. See figure 47, p. 34

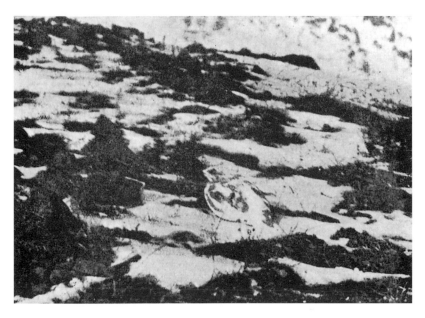

Figure 90
The camouflage effect of dappling in perfection. Total segregation of the animal's form into patterns in its environment. The outline of the animal disappears; dark holes where the snow has melted and the snowy patches of its environment merge seamlessly across its body. (Ptarmigan from the Rocky Mountains of North America, in transitional plumage. From Thayer; see footnote 51.)

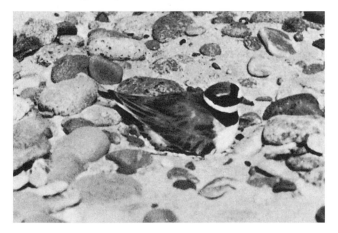

Figure 91
With the ringed plover brooding in the pebbles of the beach, the neck ring and the forehead spot are especially important for camouflage; they divide the figure of the animal into pieces that are rather roundish and resemble the pebbles. (From O. and A. Koehler: *Brütende Sandregenpfeifer. Natur und Volk* 65, 1935.)

47. Just as there the bold black bars make the delicate boundaries of the faded spot invisible, gaudy boundaries on an animal's pelt can blind the eye for the contour of the animal if it is sufficiently subdued. This effect can be observed in pure form (without accompanying disintegration), for example, in the prominent spots (eyes, etc.) on the wings of some butterflies. It can be demonstrated with simulated experiments using cardboard butterflies with the method of figure 47.[51] The contour of such a model, which can still barely be seen on a similarly colored background, disappears when you add a few brightly colored spots.

2.   THE LAW OF GOOD CONTINUATION[52]   In one of our earlier puzzle pictures, figure 20, three unfamiliar line contours were seen rather than a "4". As in that drawing, aside from the same coloration of spots, smooth continuous curves often serve as camouflage in the animal kingdom to destroy the unity of the animal's outline for the eye, and also produce false groupings with parts of the environment. The stripes of animals who live in the grass, among branches and reeds, often function as parts of longer continuous lines, exactly as the parts of the "4" in our figure 20 (compare figures 92–94). The stark lines of some butterfly pupae that hang in cracked bark often have the same effect. Other animals, such as caterpillars and stick insects, that themselves resemble a line, settle on grass stalks and similar small plant parts, so that their whole body becomes invisible by being continued on one end or the other (figure 95), like pieces of the "4". Stemlike beetles and grasshoppers stretch out their legs straight forward and backward so that they also fit perfectly into the linear background (figures 95A–D).

3.   REVERSAL OF FIGURE AND GROUND[53]   If one can make letters and all sorts of practical items disappear by assigning them the role of ground, one should assume that such an effective camouflage technique would also be used in the animal kingdom. In our previous animal examples, a part of their patterns did indeed often work as interspace, or extended background, respectively (butterfly figure 75, skunk figure

---

51. G. H. and A. H. Thayer: *Concealing Coloration in the Animal Kingdom*, New York 1902. This is the ground-breaking and most encompassing work on camouflage in the animal kingdom. Its figures addressing this special question correspond to our figure 47.

52. See p. 17 section 2.

53. See p. 1 section 1.

Figures 92–94

Camouflage through the law of good continuation (*Natur und Volk* 65, p. 253ff., figure 20).

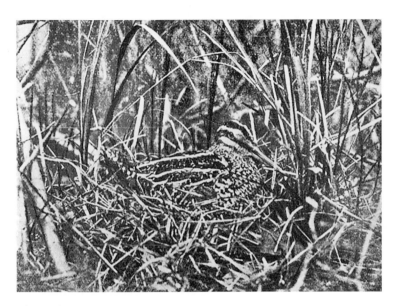

Figure 92

The American woodcock (*Gallinago wilsoni*) brooding in the bulrush undergrowth. Note, for example, how one of the stems at bottom right appears to continue through the beak to beyond the back of the head. (From Thayer; see footnote 51.)

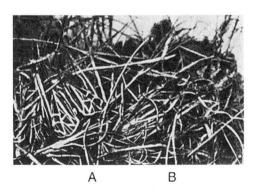

A   B

Figure 93

Two woolly bear butterflies (*Apantheles proxima*) in dry grass. Here too it is hardly possible to distinguish a grass stalk from a wing stripe, especially in the butterfly to the right above the B. (From Thayer; see footnote 51.)

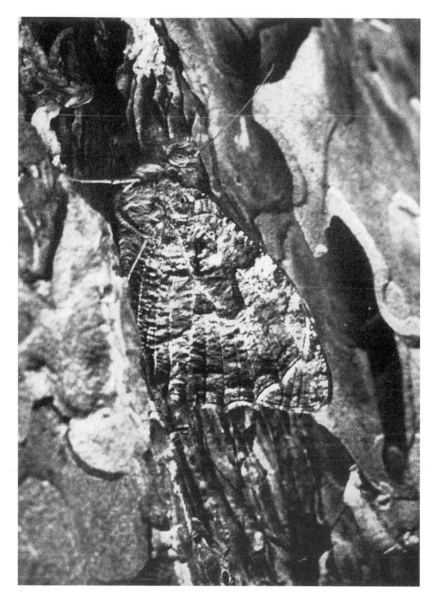

Figure 93A

Grayling on tree bark, enlarged $2\frac{1}{2}$ times. Aside from the coloration and the weathered, dusty appearance, continuous lines are effective in the most astonishing way. From the bottom upward the splintery fissure of the bark continues into the fine wing veins. From above right, the arched edges of the protruding bark flakes merge seamlessly with the diagonal contours across the wings. Not only the border itself, but also its shadow, repeats itself in tracings of the wings so exactly, that the lower half seems actually to be separated from the upper. (From A. Seitz: *Semele. Natur und Volk* 64, 1934.)

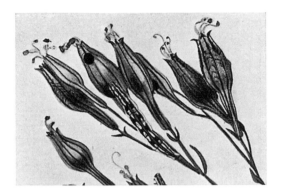

Figure 94
Looper (*Eupithecia schiefereri* BOH., France) in a wild flax umbel. Depending on the brightness of the background, for the eye either the bright stripes become continuations of the plant parts above and below them and the dark stripes parts of the background, or vice versa. One readily realizes that the stripes do not function in the sense of similarity in general (section 2): if the caterpillar sat crosswise to the umbel, its stripes would no longer have a camouflage effect, unless they themselves ran across the caterpillar's body, so that they would again continue roughly in a straight line with adjoining parts of the plant. (From Dietze; see text for figure 75.)

86, caterpillar figure 94). But there is an opportunity for smaller creatures, especially those that are long and thin, and that live in small furrows, cracks, or crevices, to become entirely a *gap* to the observer's eye, and thus become invisible like the pencil in figure 5. According to Thayer's conjecture, the glittering black color of some young water fowl may make one believe instead of seeing the bird that one is seeing through the reeds into dark, glistening water.

7. OVERVIEW

There is hardly a law of vision that is not found again serving camouflage in the animal kingdom. In reviewing them, however, one of the most significant and widely used principles of camouflage remains that we have not touched on, because we are not yet familiar with the psychological prerequisites of its effect.

Let us now go back and review figures 2, 16, 20, and 29 once again and recall the first impressions they made.[54] Now we can appreciate how

---

54. See pp. 2, 13, 17, 21.

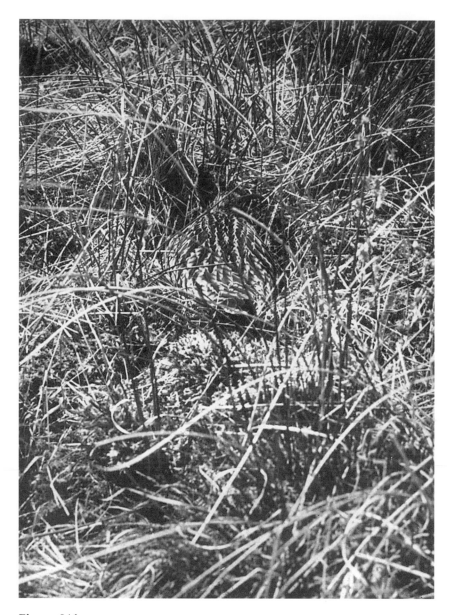

Figure 94A

The Eurasian curlew on its nest. Stems and their interspaces appear to continue over the back of the animal; its shape is thereby resolved completely into parts of the environment, but only as long as it does not move. With any movement it would immediately pop out from its environment according to the law of common fate. As if the animal knew this, it sits motionless between the stalks, until one almost touches it, whereas in any other environment it would long before have taken flight. (Photo: Fischer, Braunschweig.)

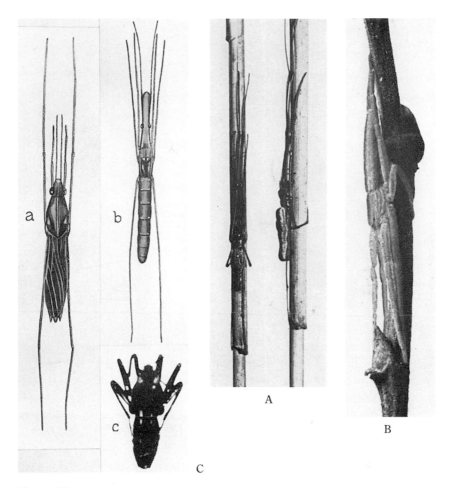

Figure 95
Protective posture according to the law of good continuation. A and B in the natural environment, C removed from it. Only with C could one think that the similarity to a stick would fool a predator into ignoring that what it sees lying there is an animal. As A (esp. left) and B reveal, the predator should not see a little stick in place of the animal, but rather nothing at all, according to the law of good continuation. A. Stretch spider (*Tetragnatha solandrii*). In this position (according to Steiniger's findings) the spider becomes hard or even impossible to detect even by its natural enemies such as robins. B. Slender crab spider (*Tibellus oblongus*). (C-a) Waterstrider (*Limnoporus rufoscutellatus*), (C-b) water measurer (*Hydrometra stagnorum*). (C-c) The watercricket (*Velia currens*) assumes a different posture; with its rounded body the stretched-out posture would be pointless. (Figures 95 A–C from Steiniger: *Natur und Museum*, 1933, p. 368, and *Natur und Volk* pp. 18–20, 1936.)

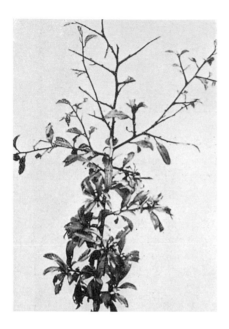

Figure 95D
Again, camouflage according to the law of good continuation. Animals that already look like a narrow stripe need only worry about a proper elongated posture of their bodies. The caterpillar of the rare swallow-tailed butterfly (*Papilio podalirius*) on a blackthorn branch. Compare also figure 94. (From Süffert: *Phänomene visueller Anpassung. Z. Morph. Ök. Tiere* 26, pp. 148–316, 1932.)

it happens with the hunter when a long-sought animal suddenly, magically appears before him. We now realize that it is wrong to say that the animal was previously poorly visible. In fact, the observer saw, circumstances permitting, quite clearly at the respective spot, but unfortunately saw only things that were quite different from what he was looking for. He could not see what he was looking for until a real change occurred in his visual field by which the shapes seen initially had themselves become partly invisible. Perhaps the examples of camouflage also may have made our assertion in chapter 3[55] more plausible. Even with open, healthy eyes and in sufficient lighting, it is not at all self-evident that we actually see *things that are present* in our environment, instead of the most fantastic phantoms. We are blind even to the most familiar things, when their perceived boundaries are deflected by their color and markings (and the color and markings of their surround), in accordance with psychological laws, from the location or only orientation[56] of the actual outlines.

---

55. See p. 39f.
56. See p. 6f.

6

BRIGHTNESS AND SPATIAL FORM

1. THE BUMPY ROAD

Anyone who has driven in an automobile at night will surely have had the following odd experience. In front of the car in the beams of the headlights stretches a landscape that appears more like a hilly landscape than a flat road, yet the car drives just as smoothly forward on it as on any ordinary road. This is nothing unusual, if you are well acquainted with the road and know that it has a well-maintained and relatively even surface. When an oncoming car appears from the darkness ahead, suddenly the road becomes covered with wavy undulations (figure 96).

There is no question that these undulations correspond to real small bumps on the road, it is just that they seem extremely exaggerated. How is that? Under street lamps the highway does not look less flat than it does in daylight; it appears most bumpy when there is no other light source in the area except for the headlights of a car. But even the beams of the headlights do not make everything that they touch appear uneven. When leaving the driveway they shine on the wall of the house ahead almost at right angles. The wall does not look less flat in the glaring headlights than in broad daylight. The wavy effect must therefore be due to the unusual direction with which the beams of the headlights strike the surface of the road. They strike it at a glancing angle that is nearly parallel to the surface.

2. GLANCING LIGHT BETRAYS HIDDEN IRREGULARITIES

Illuminating a surface from a glancing angle can bring out tiny surface irregularities that are too small to be detected with binocular (so-called stereoscopic) vision. Thus words written in pencil that have been fully erased become clearly readable again in tangential light (as long as they were not written too lightly). The tiny impressed groove made by the pencil point in the paper can then be seen, even though in normal light

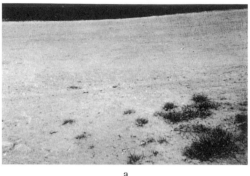

a

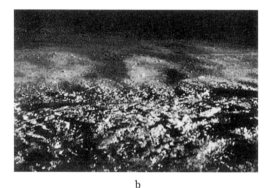

b

Figure 96
Two views of the same stretch of road, seen from the same point. (Note the grass tuft lower right.) (a) In scattered daylight it looks beautifully smooth and even, not just here in the picture, but also in reality with binocular vision. (b) At night in the headlights. You would think that there must have been an earthquake that meanwhile changed the flat surface of the road into a hilly landscape. The difference with binocular viewing of the actual street is no less than in the picture.

it remains completely invisible. And it is seen not just as a dark line on the shadowed side accompanied by a bright line on the light side, but perfectly clear and compelling in spatial depth. There is really only one possible error here: namely, that you can sometimes see the groove as an *elevation*, a *ridge*, instead of as a groove (figure 97). Similarly, it is often possible to read typewritten letters from the back of a sheet in tangential light, even when no trace of the ink shines through. You can see distinctly delineated and clearly formed elevations, where in scattered light there is nothing, or only a blurred bright glimmer (figure 98). The fine grain, fibers, and texture of completely uniformly colored papers are also

Figures 97 and 98

Completely colorless writing tracks in paper that in diffuse light (a) are invisible, or are visible only as blurred bright spots, emerge as sharp and clear in tangential light (b). The difference is in reality no less than in the photos.

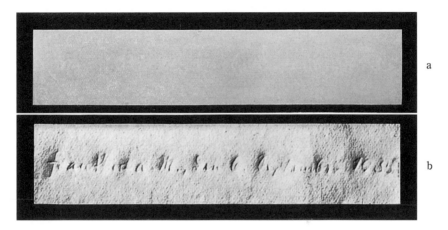

Figure 97

Pencil tracks. The fact that it really is the same piece of paper can perhaps be seen most easily from the number 6.

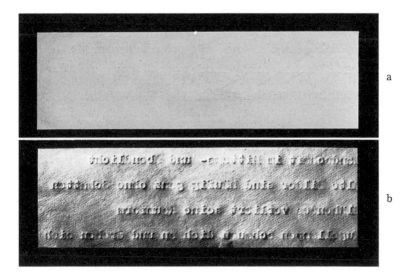

Figure 98

A piece of a typewritten page, seen from the back.

brought out if they are not too rough—not so much by the effect of binocular vision as through the effect of the glancing light. In vertical or scattered light those textures disappear even in binocular vision, when differences in elevation are in fact sufficiently large—according to the theory—to be noticeable in binocular vision (figure 99).

It is the same with solid bodies, which, because of their great distance, project identical retinal images to both eyes as only flat objects do nearby. At short range and under favorable conditions, the binocular system can perceive astonishingly fine depth differences because of variations between the two retinal images of the same object. But with increasing distance this capability, for external reasons, falls off much more quickly than one generally imagines. *Depth acuity* is defined as the smallest difference in depth that can just be discriminated under optimal conditions from a given distance. At 1 meter's distance the depth acuity is still about 0.5 mm, at 50 meters it is 1 m, at 500 meters distance it is already over 100 m, and beyond 2.5 km even infinitely large differences of distance are imperceptible for the binocular system. This means that if space perception depended solely on the interaction between the eyes, the most corpulent gentleman at 50 m, the most impressive country estate at 500 m, and also the mightiest mountain range and the most powerful thunder cloud beyond 1000 m should look no different than cardboard scenery.

It is at that range that the effect of light and shadow becomes especially important. This is why mountain landscapes around noontime often look somewhat boring and lifeless, sometimes really almost like stage sets, especially in perfectly clear or uniformly overcast weather. Experienced photographers therefore take pictures of such areas only in the oblique light of the morning or evening (figure 100), at least when they are interested not in a particular mood, but in the clarity of the landscape features, if possible not in the direction of the sun's rays. For the same reason it looks on all pictures of the moon as if mountain ranges were only to be found on the shadowy border (figure 101), whereas on the full moon, even with the best telescope, all you see are bright spots rather than elevations, as on the right of figure 101.

3.   UNIFORM BRIGHTNESS HIDES EVEN TANGIBLE SPATIAL FORM IN OUR IMMEDIATE NEIGHBORHOOD

In the preceding examples, cues for binocular vision are missing, and illumination steps in helpfully by creating unusually strong brightness dif-

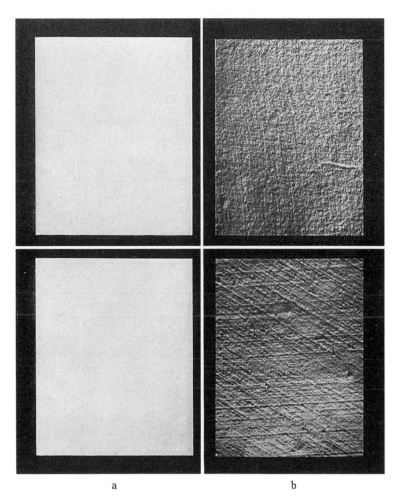

a   b

Figure 99

Japanese papers, which look flat in diffuse light (a) and can scarcely be distinguished, show unevenness of an entirely different kind in tangential light (b). Nonetheless, one cannot say that glancing light correctly portrays the paper. For example, wartlike elevations on the lower paper, which in part look almost as high as they are wide, are in reality significantly flatter. Their height measures approximately $\frac{1}{10}$ to $\frac{1}{5}$ mm, in parts certainly still less. That it is in each case precisely the same piece of paper can be seen in the upper pair from the thicker horizontal fiber to the right slightly below center, and from the small bulge at the lower left in the lower pair from the slightly bowed, diagonal fiber in the middle of the left border.

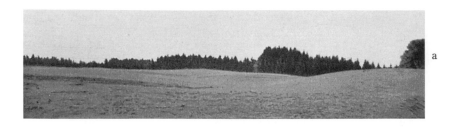

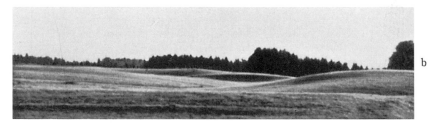

Figure 100
The same meadowlands photographed at (a) noon and (b) in the evening. Where one only sees monotonous flat rising ground at noon, in the evening sun peculiar slopes appear with rather sharply delineated borders. (Photo: Gertrud Kautzsch, Hohenschäftlarn b. München.)

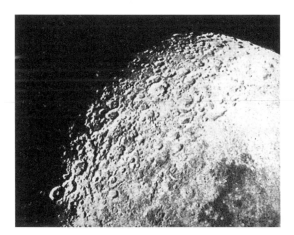

Figure 101
South pole region of the moon. Only at the shadowed border, that is, as seen from the moon in twilight, does an extraordinary tumult of craters appear. To the right, where it is broad daylight on the moon, one sees only hazy white spots, although those regions contain mountain ranges that are no lower and no less rugged. On the full moon one sees the least through a telescope, for then everything on the face of the moon looks like the right-hand part of our photo. (From Bruno Bürgel: *Aus fernen Welten*. Berlin, 1911.)

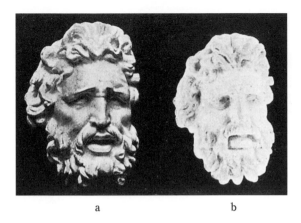

a   b

Figure 102
The same figure (head of Zeus) in different illuminations. (a) In soft light coming mainly from the upper left, the bodily shapes are worked out most finely and clearly for the eye. (With such a sculpture a glancing light that emanates from one single point is naturally not the best. The shadow side of the face would disappear in it, like the shadow side of the moon in the sun's light. (b) In very diffuse, slightly stronger light from below right. The bodily shapes are dull, blurred, and lifeless, almost entirely flattened—even in reality. Nonetheless, there are recent books about sculpture that lack the words illumination, light, and shade in their index. (Figures 102, 103, and 105 from Luckiesh: *Light and Shade and Their Applications.* New York, 1916.)

ferences. But illumination can severely disturb binocular vision even in its own domain, when it works in the opposite sense; that is, when it actually weakens or eliminates brightness differences. It is no accident that it is a difficult task to display sculptures in the right light, so that their volumetric form becomes visible in all its liveliness and delicacy. In light that is too diffuse and uniform, the volumetric form becomes dull and blurred, and in reality hardly less than in figures 102 and 103.

The brightness of a monochromatic object's surface appears most uniform when you make the object itself glow. For example, the key in figure 104 seems to lose its volumetric shape as it begins to glow red hot. If you have access to rooms with globe lamps made of translucent milky glass, you can easily try a similar experiment yourself. All you need to do is to turn the light on and off. Naturally, the globe must be well cleaned inside and out and have a frosted glass light bulb, so that no shadows of the filament fall on the globe from inside. As soon as the light is turned *on* the globe light *loses its curvature* (and its shininess) and seemingly becomes a flat disk. This is most noticeable when only one of two adjacent lamps is lit. Since the apparent disk is never distorted by

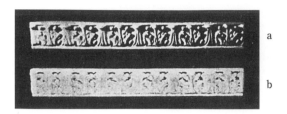

Figure 103
The same frieze of letters. (a) In glancing, slightly diagonal lighting from above, it stands out clearly and strongly. (b) In diffuse light coming predominantly from below, it appears vague and blurred, partially invisible.

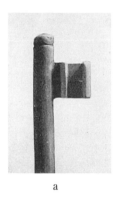 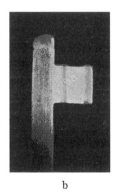

a   b

Figure 104
In direct daylight the sharply delineated shape of the key (a) becomes more vague the stronger the key glows, and indeed long before one is blinded by its glow. The real reason is that with strong glow its surface becomes almost uniformly bright (b).

perspective, it is always turned exactly toward the observer, and as you move about, it seems to turn to always face toward you. If you walk along a row of such lamps, they seem to follow you, like the heads of a line of soldiers that follow their commander as he paces in front of them. Dust and houseflies of course keep this ghostly experience from being all too familiar. In figure 105b the uniform brightness of the lower globe is achieved by scattered light that falls on it from the outside. But the effect is the same as with the self-luminous globe lamp. You really cannot distinguish the globe from the flat disk above, whereas with light from a window (figure 105a), its surface looks just as rounded as its circular outline.

      Even in real life the globe does not look any more convex than the one in the picture. The reason for this is quite simple, although it is not

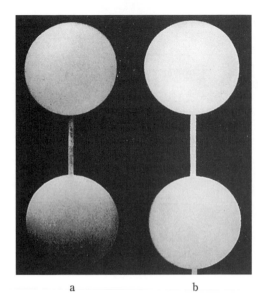

a   b

Figure 105
The same disk and globe (a) in direct, slightly diffuse illumination and (b) in completely diffuse light. A uniformly colored globe, with neither highlight nor shadowed side—even in real life—cannot be distinguished from a flat disk. (From Luckiesh; see figure 102.)

easy to discover. A globe whose surface has no texture and no imperfections offers the two eyes no depth cues of any kind. In order to produce the impression of depth differences, stereo vision requires *sharp points* or *lines*. The only sharp line on the uniformly colored globe, however, is its *outline*. And its image is just as round in both eyes, just like the image of a uniformly colored flat disk in the frontoparallel plane, so no stereo effect can occur on the globe under these conditions. When a uniformly colored globe does appear correctly convex, it is the distribution of light and shadow that is the only cause of this effect. In the following discussion we will address only this immediate spatial effect of the brightness distribution.

4. AN OFTEN REPEATED BUT FALSE EXPLANATION: SEEN AND DEDUCED DEPTH

How do differences of slope originate from differences of brightness? No one I have ever asked this question has yet been at a loss for an answer. "I do not see the depth relationships at all," is about what one says, "I only infer them, that is, I imagine them. In reality I see only light and shadow. But I know how to deal with this, and based on that knowledge I can interpret the brightness relations as depth. When I assume that an object (real or depicted) is illuminated from one side, say the left, then it goes without saying that the brighter portions must be oriented toward

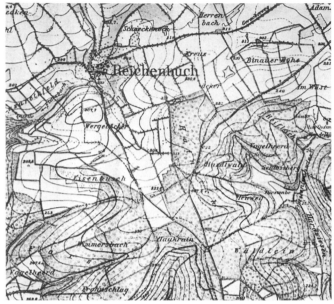

Fig. 106a

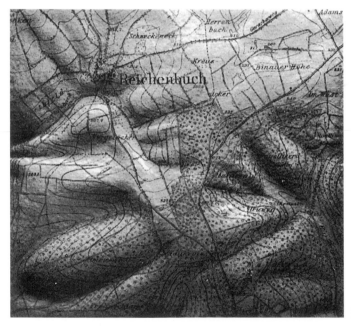

Fig. 106b

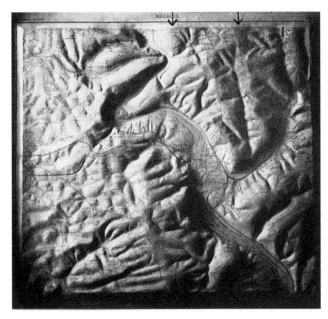

Fig. 106c

Figure 106

(a) Section of the Baden topographical map, sheet 34, Mosbach. Elevations are indicated by contour lines and can be very exactly deduced through these. But they are not actually seen. In some places, for example, the forest valley at the lower right, one does indeed see a little of the slope of the land, but contour lines alone are not responsible. Through the varying density of the sketched forest a kind of shading arises, and this is the main cause of the depth impression. (b) The same map section in a Wenschow relief picture, illuminated rather exactly from the upper border (that is, on the map, from the north). Here you can see the elevations effortlessly without having to think about anything. (c) The relief map, out of whose upper border (between the two arrows) figure 106b was cut out illuminated from the left (a little from above). The contour lines are invisible, and yet the spatial effect is undiminished.

the light, thus, for example, oriented to the left, and the darker portions oriented away from the light, in our example toward the right."

In some circumstances you actually think such thoughts. But truth be told, who, in any one of the previous figures, remembers having at first noticed only the brightness differences, and having inferred the spatial form after the fact by reasoning? Since this is a rather delicate question, which has lured even the most famous scholars to excuses, we would rather first like to present a new example to clarify the difference between *seeing and imagining*, an issue that has become completely obliterated by philosophical and psychological treatises of the last two centuries.

There are different ways of indicating in a picture that the depicted object should have differences in elevation. On maps, for example, you make use of contour lines from whose direction and density you can deduce the slope of the land quite precisely, as long as you know that water is not found on mountain peaks but in valleys. But you can only see the slope directly where the contour lines are especially dense, as in figure 106a bottom right (naturally there is already a kind of shading just from the different density of the sketched forest texture). Compare with this the impression of the relief map illuminated by *glancing illumination* (figure 106b). Here the slopes and differences in elevation of the landscape are simply there. You just need to open your eyes and you *see* them without racking your brains about it. In figure 106b you do indeed see the contour lines as well, but they are quite irrelevant for the spatial impression. This is evident in figure 106c, where the contour lines are absent, and yet the impression of a mountain landscape is undiminished.

The two relief maps can also serve to eliminate a similar misunderstanding. Figures 106b and 106c look without any doubt far more mountainous than figure 106a. But that does not mean that what you see there as elevations is any more reliable in its details than what you can infer from them in figure 106a. Thus the valley that runs approximately north-south on the lower right in figure 106b seems too flat relative to the others, as does the side valley in 106c, which leads in an exactly westerly direction down toward the main river (the same valley that strikes the middle of the left border at right angles in figure 106b). This occurs with every valley that happens by chance to run parallel to the direction of illumination. The spatial interpretation of contour lines is independent of such chance alignments, so replacing contour lines with shading would be foolish.

5. THE EVIDENCE OF EVOLUTIONARY HISTORY

Do you really see the brightness differences that bring out the impression of depth as precisely as the above explanation assumes? The development of painting throughout human history, as well as throughout the life of the individual, proves the opposite; namely, that from beginning to end, you do indeed see very precisely whether an object is made of black, gray, or white material, or is painted with these colors. But you

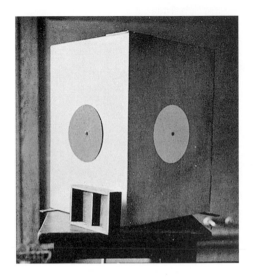

Figure 107

Which of the two disks is brighter—the dark gray one on the left or the white one on the right? As you can see, the dark gray one is under bright illumination, the white one in shadow. But with only two small holes in an occluding overlay sheet you can also see that because of different illumination, the dark gray disk is actually brighter; that is, it reflects more light into the eye than the white one. In this illustration in addition to the separation of illumination and surface color, there is effectively an analogous contrast change of the surrounds on the round disks (compare chapter 8). This effect, however, can be eliminated in the experiment.

only see very imprecisely how brightly it happens to be illuminated, and you do not see at all the strength of the illuminating light that is reflected from its various places and that reaches the eye. But it would be exactly the latter that would be of significance if a spatial inference is to have any success.

No children ever think of shading their pictures without a model, or instruction on how to achieve a depth effect, even if they notice and regret the lack of spatial depth in their picture. "I remember very well from my childhood years that shading in a drawing seemed an unjustified and distorted style to me, and that a contour drawing seemed to me much more satisfactory," reported Ernst Mach.[57] I too have an unforgettable memory of the class when our drawing instructor explained to us 13- to 14-year-old boys that to produce the impression of a black suit correctly, one must paint the black cloth facing toward the window brighter than the snow-white collar on the shadowed side. Even an adult cannot see this without using special tricks. In figure 107 you see two circular disks, the left disk made of dark gray paper, the right disk of white. The figure depicts this condition, except that in reality the left paper looks much darker than shown in the illustration. However, it

---

57. *Die Analyse der Empfindungen*, 9th ed. Jena, 1922, p. 171.

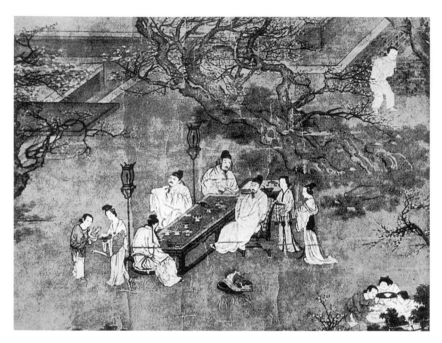

Figure 108
A painting masterpiece without the slightest hint of light and shadow. Detail of
Spring Feast by Ch'ou Ying, China, ca. 1500. (From Otto Fischer: *Chinesische Land-
schaftsmalerei.* Munich, 1923.)

also corresponds to the facts that in the illumination prevailing in the illustration, the dark gray (left) disk actually is "brighter" than the white
(right) one; it is sending a stronger light into the eye than the right one.
But even the most practiced photographer can see this only by laying a
piece of uniform paper with two small holes on the picture, so that
nothing but a small sector of each circular disk is visible. The peculiar
and physically inexplicable impression that even deeply shadowed surfaces can appear white, while brightly lit surfaces can appear to be black,
is known in psychology as *brightness constancy*. Originally it was believed
that this impressive phenomenon should not be taken too seriously, and
it too was explained as knowledge on the basis of logical inference, or
reasoning—until it was discovered that the phenomenon works not
only for people, but that it is equally true for chickens, whose primitive
brain is surely incapable of such deliberations. For example, a chicken
that is offered a white kind of grain that tastes good and a dark (or
blue) grain that tastes bad, both grains being always offered in bright

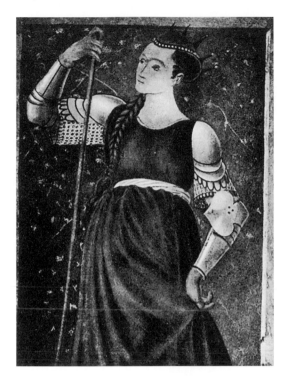

Figure 109
Early Italian painting in which shading is used to indicate roundness (arms, folds of clothing), but only in parts; for example, not at all on the head and neck. Castagno *Tomyris* (detail) fresco, about 1450, Florence, Cenacolo di Santa Apollonia. (From Hausenstein: *Die Malerei der frühen Italiener*. Munich, 1922.)

sunlight, after training always chooses the white grains without hesitation. This holds true even when the grains are presented in the shade (or in blue light) and thereby reflect the same weak, or even weaker (or equally blue) light into the eyes as the disliked dark (or blue) grains presented nearby in bright sunlight that the chicken has not touched for quite a while.

Not only unschooled children, but even the greatest artists from the Stone Age onward for millennia have ignored differences of illumination in their paintings. In East Asia the practice continues to this day (figure 108), except when trying to imitate European painting. Even in Europe illumination was ignored until the beginning of modern times. And when artists did attempt to indicate the roundness of the body, folds of drapery, and the like by shading, it was much too weak and full

Figures 110 and 111
Two portraits from the same era, with opposite interpretations. (From Esswein and
Hausenstein: *Das deutsche Bild des 16. Jahrhunderts*. Munich, 1923.)

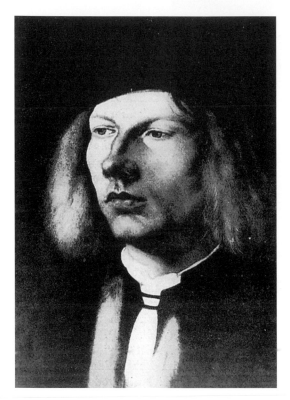

Figure 110
Doubtless the tangible, physical is deliberately emphasized in this worldly represen-
tation through exaggeration of brightness differences with side illumination. Albrecht
Dürer, died 1528, *Portrait of a Young Man* (detail), Hampton Court Castle.

of contradictions, especially in the distribution of light and shadow,
compared with reality (figure 109). It is remarkable that even in times
when the correct representation of light and shadow was known, in
sixteenth-century Germany, renowned artists avoided it or at least did
not make use of it with certain objects, for example, in portraits. In
children's drawings, cave paintings of the Stone Age, Egyptian frescoes,
and Byzantine mosaics it is possible to ascribe the lack of shading to lack
of ability, or at least this interpretation cannot be refuted. But with
artists (e.g., Hans Baldung) who in other respects must be counted as

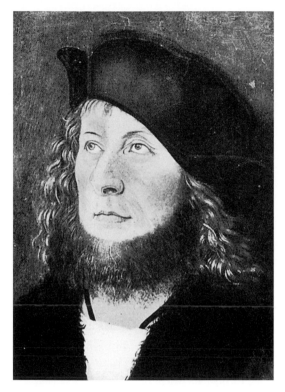

Figure 111
The solid volumetric form is not valued in its own right, it is only hinted at to the
extent that is necessary to make the character visible; the light is diffuse, the shadows
a mere hint. Ascribed to Martin Schaffner, died 1541, portrait (detail), Hanover,
Provincial Museum.

belonging to very progressive movements of their time, the decision not
to use shading can only have been a matter of judgment of highest art-
istry. The decision was whether the face of a man should be seen
primarily as something that fills a certain space and that one can touch
with one's hands, or as reflecting a certain essence and spiritual attitude
(figures 110 and 111).

6.   The Spatial Effect of Brightness Is Just as Immediate and
Primary as that of Binocular Vision

Contrasts of light and shadow are extremely important to create a sense
of depth, and often are its only cue. Nevertheless it is totally wrong to

suggest that in this case brightness contrasts are what you see first, and that it is only gradually through experience that you learn to interpret them spatially. Instead, you immediately see elevations and depressions of bodily structures in shadowed areas of the visual field. This is a consequence of a mysterious process of transformation that occurs somewhere along the way from the neural excitation of the retinas to the seat of vision in the brain. If you become aware of the shadows at all, you might consider them the inevitable but insignificant consequence of the interaction of light and form. It is only relatively late in their training that some people, who engage this issue more thoroughly as artists or researchers, discover that it is not only with pictures, but also with real objects that the bulges and depressions on an object would often be invisible if the brightness differences were missing.

The emergence of depth from shading cues is no more miraculous than the emergence from two flat retinal images of the perceived world that extends in depth as well as in height and width. In fact, most people die without ever having experienced anything of the existence of the two flat retinal images. Even though natural scientists know about them, they cannot see them any more in their own experience than anyone else. How these transformations actually occur and why they occur exactly as they do—namely, in a way that is so useful in most cases—and not entirely differently, is still unknown. But evidence suggests that we will understand these issues in brightness perception sooner than in binocular vision, despite the untiring work that has been dedicated to its study for a century.

7

Gestalt Laws in the Spatial Effect of Perspective Drawings

Most of us would consider it rather audacious to assert that in vision there could be still more spatial cues that might be just as immediate and primary as those of binocular vision. But according to research of recent years we have good reason to assume that this applies not only to the distribution of brightness, but furthermore to almost everything else that today falls under the heading of empirical depth criteria, that is, cues to depth based on experience.

1. Are Perspective Drawings Interpreted as Having Depth?

Consider, for instance, perspective interpretation of flat line drawings. What is it that should be interpreted there and what should be the result of such interpretation? First, differences in size should be reinterpreted as differences in distance (figure 112), and second, certain angular relationships and differences in height and width (foreshortening) should be interpreted as sloping configurations in depth. And that should occur not only for drawings, but also for real things, such as when observing them with only one eye. But just as with the effect of light and shadow, this theory also falls apart in the face of the evidence of developmental history.

Generally we see, to be sure, quite precisely whether the objects in our environment are bounded *by right-angled or oblique-angled surfaces*. We never confuse a round cake platter with an elliptical meat platter, even though the cake platter is always imaged as elliptical in the eye, except when we look straight down on it from above. We would never judge a young boy standing next to us as larger than a man on the other side of the street. We can occlude cupboards, houses, and entire villages with our thumb, if we hold it up close to one eye (with the other eye closed); and even then our thumb does not seem much larger than usual. Most of the time we also see very clearly which objects are closer and which are farther away, and whether they are standing in front of us straight

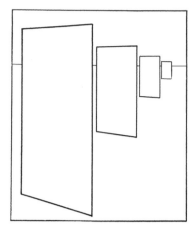

Figure 112
Depth effect of size differences and of distortion. Instead of a row of differently sized, asymmetrical trapezoids that lie next to each other at different heights in the plane of the drawing, one sees equally sized rectangular slabs that stand out at the same height and are equally spaced in depth.

Figures 113
Depth effect of oblique angles. You do not see parallelograms drawn superimposed on the paper's surface, but rather a cube (a) and a roof (b, c). The drawing contains only oblique angles, but you see only right angles (the one exception is the crease in the roof in c). (Figures 113, 115, 116a–g, 117–119, 121–128 from H. Kopfermann: *Psychologische Untersuchungen über die Wirkung zweidimensionaler Darstellungen körperlicher Gebilde. Psychol. Forschg.* 13, 1930.)

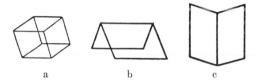

a   b   c

and vertical, or sloping in depth. That we usually cannot specify the configuration precisely in meters or degrees of angle is beside the point.

As for those essential cues without which perspective interpretation would be impossible, that is, distortions and foreshortenings, the situation is even worse. Children (as well as naive adults) usually do not notice those distortions in actual objects (figures 113a and b). If someone had explained to us after we had gone through the world for twelve years with open eyes, that we actually see things the way they project on the retina, we would have been utterly surprised and astonished. But even after we have accepted the arguments of the art teacher and made them our own, we are still a long way from being able to see things as he wishes. Ask an acquaintance to sketch a plate on the table in perspective,

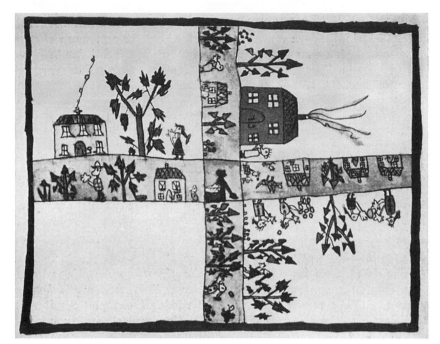

Fig. 113A

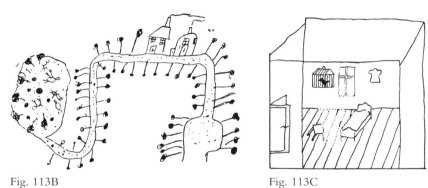

Fig. 113B   Fig. 113C

Figures 113A–C

The fact that the path to the playground is equally wide everywhere, and that the streets intersect at right angles, and that the houses and trees stand vertically at the edges of the path, are facts that we not only know, but that we actually see despite the distortions of the retinal image; and so the child draws it this way. The drawer of 113A attempted furthermore to capture the fact that the houses and trees on the opposite sides of a street rise in the same direction. (A) Street crossing drawn by a 10-year-old. (From G. Britsch: *Theorie der bildenden Kunst.* Munich, 1926.) (B) (below left). Snowball fight drawn by a 9-year-old. (From Kerschensteiner: *Die Entwicklung der zeichnerischen Begabung.* Munich, 1905.) (C) Perspective drawing by a 12-year-old. It deviates considerably from the retinal image: transparent ceiling; door suspended in the air; floor with parallel grooves, occluded by both side walls; bird cage depicted entirely face-on. (In the dotted areas there were people in the original drawing. Universalhist. Inst. Leipzig.)

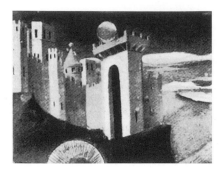

Figure 114
Early Italian painting with still very uncertain and inconsistent perspective. Detail of an altar painting by Fra Angelico, died 1455, Florence, San Marco. (From Hausenstein: *Die Malerei der frühen Italiener*. Munich, 1922.)

without sighting it first by the artist's "thumb-and-pencil" method. Unless he is very practiced, the ellipse always turns out to be too much like a circle. Or you walk, let us say, from a distance of four meters to a distance of one meter toward an acquaintance and ask him how much taller you now appear to him. If he does not calculate the answer, he might perhaps say one and a half times or at most twice as tall, and never imagine that the perspective enlargement actually amounts to 1:4 (compare also figure 113C).

The history of art also confirms this finding. If you wish to portray houses and larger objects halfway recognizably on a flat drawing surface, without either omitting something essential or severing the spatial relationships, you must, whether you like it or not, depict the edges running into the background as slanting lines. But how late in life did you learn, and at the expense of how many computational and mechanical expedients (figures 114A and B), to execute these slanting lines correctly? Consider also how narrow the circle is within the fine arts, within which this kind of correctness was valued at all (compare figures 114 and also 108); and generally how little the mastery of perspective representation has to do with true artistic merit even within this circle—the European painting of the sixteenth to nineteenth centuries.

But if the cues to depth are so hard to discover and so uncertain, and when as a rule they are understood so grossly wrong, if at all, how should you be able to infer anything reliable from them? You might just as well expect that someone would be able to translate Greek manuscripts before becoming acquainted with Greek letters.[58]

---

58. The fact that we overlook typographical errors and thus recognize the meaning of words without first identifying each individual letter, is no counter-evidence. That kind of recognition occurs only when there are a few false or illegible letters among very many correct ones, not when just about everything is wrong or illegible.

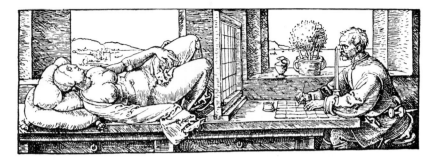

Figure 114A
Sighting device. Between the eye and the object stands a glass pane with a square grid etched on it. Directly in front of the eye there is a pointed sight firmly fastened to the table. Through appropriate head movements the tip of the sight is successively aligned with various points of the display, and it is determined where in the square grid the superposition occurs. The located point is entered on the second square grid that lies on the table.

2.   THE CONSTANCY OF THE SHAPE AND SIZE OF SEEN OBJECTS[*]

So we are confronted again with the same puzzle as with brightness. Two things that are imaged in the eye as completely different sizes can nonetheless look equally large. A solid body whose image on the retina takes on the most diverse shapes with rotation or through a change in viewpoint, nevertheless looks completely unchanged, except for certain limiting cases. Perceptually it appears as a stable, shape-invariant object, not some rubbery elastic thing, as you might expect from what we know about the image on the retina.

In other words, our eyes are designed such that they see the things in our immediate environment as near as possible to the right shape and the right size, not what the physicists call apparent size (and shape), that corresponds to the visual angle—which is what you would see if you looked at your own retina. But one does not do that. To convince yourself of this conclusively, you need only to generate a retinal image of constant retinal size (and shape). For this purpose, you can form an after-image, for example, by looking for ten to twenty seconds from some distance steadily into the middle of a small bright window or a light bulb (not an arc lamp!). If you then look first at a distant wall, the dark

---

[*] Translators' note: There is no section 2 in the German text; sections have been relabeled.

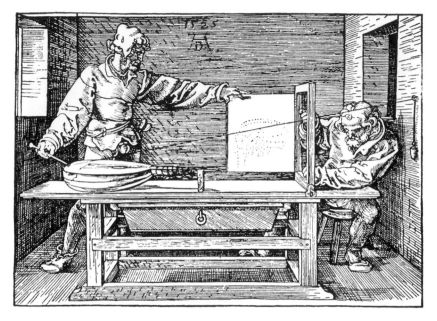

Figure 114B
Measuring device. In this case the "artist" need not look at what he produces; he just
needs to read the scales, his equipment does the rest. The eye is replaced by a ring on
the wall, the viewing direction or line of sight by a piece of string. The fixation
point is replaced by the point of a rod attached to the string. The string runs loosely
through the ring and is held taut by a weight. Between the eye [ring] and the model
is a frame the size of the picture that records the projection. Individual points of the
model are scanned one by one with the fixation point [rod]. For each point on the
model, a point is marked where the line of sight [string] passes through the plane of
the frame, and those points are transferred one by one to the recording picture. (Figures 114A and B from Dürer's *Unterweisung der Messung*.)

afterimage there appears much larger than the original stimulus, whereas
on a piece of paper held in your hand, it becomes so small that you
might have trouble seeing it at first. If you move the paper back and
forth in depth, you can see the afterimage positively grow and shrink,[59]
all with a single fixed retinal image. It is also noteworthy how unexpectedly distorted the shape of the afterimage appears if you had been standing at an angle to the window that served as the stimulus, but then view
the afterimage straight against a wall. It is hard to believe that the retinal

---

59. When the afterimage starts to become weak, one can usually refresh it somewhat
by occasional vigorous blinking of the eyelids.

Figure 115

A drawing that looks compellingly three-dimensional although the portrayed physical body, a regular six-sided (and also transparent) double pyramid, is very rare. If experience and professional knowledge were decisive, this drawing should appear so vividly spatial only to a mineralogist who has studied crystalline forms long enough for them to be familiar. Other people would be expected to see much more readily a square with all sorts of oblique lines inside its perimeter, especially on first glance.

image of the window had been as distorted as the afterimage now appears. The real apparent size, that is, the immediate size impression, therefore does not correspond to the so-called apparent size of physical optics, except in the limiting case of greatest distance, for example, with star constellations.

But since this term is not used in physical optics only for this limiting case, one should avoid the expression apparent size altogether and replace it with visual angle. The term retinal size would also be possible; but it is inappropriate, not only because this size varies with the diameter of the eyeball, but above all because in physical optics it is the *angle* that really matters.

The same holds for the amazing phenomena of size constancy and shape constancy of perceived objects despite variations of the retinal image, which also do not depend on sophisticated geometrical deliberations of the observer, as one was initially inclined to assume. For there is no longer any doubt that these constancies are already fully developed in the vision of higher animals that are surely incapable of engaging in such deliberations.[60]

3.   Effective and Ineffective Representations of Solid Bodies

Cube and roof shapes are certainly more common in our lives than such oblique-angled groups of lines as presented in figure 113, when interpreted as flat, plane patterns. A transparent, six-sided, double pyramid, however, is apt to be familiar to hardly any reader. Nonetheless we cannot resist seeing figure 115, just as figure 113, as a solid body, instead of a flat drawing.

---

60. Compare Wolfgang Köhler: *Optische Untersuchungen am Schimpansen und am Haushuhn. Verh. Preuß. Akad., Math.-Phys. Kl. 3*, 1915.

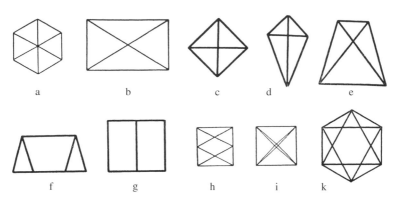

Figure 116

Drawings that do not look three-dimensional although they all are correct perspective representations of very simple and familiar solid objects: cube (a), three-sided pyramid (b, c, d, e), four-sided pyramid (c), three-edged beam or roof (f, g), four-sided double pyramid (h, i, k). The flat drawing itself is so regular that it does not pop out in the least from the paper's surface. (Figures 116 a–g from Kopfermann; see figure 113; h–k from Metzger: *Tiefenerscheinungen in optischen Bewegungsfeldern. Psychol. Forschg.* 20, 1934.)

But given the foregoing discussion, it is out of the question that we are irresistably inclined to see a solid body in any drawing that even permits that interpretation. Otherwise we would also be required to perceive the drawings in figure 116 as solid bodies, and even more so, since these all represent familiar solid shapes. However, in this case we see nothing but flat figures. Even when we make an effort to see the solid-body interpretation, we are not always successful (probably easiest still in figures 116e and k).

By contrast, it is just as hard to see the flat interpretation in figure 117 and figure 115, even though here the depicted solid bodies are certainly much less familiar than those in figure 116. You need only move the view point a tiny bit (figure 118) no longer to recognize the solid shape. More correctly, the drawings now strive as it were to act as flat images, even though they are just as valid solid-body representations as the others.

4.   EVEN THE DEPTH EFFECT OF LINE DRAWINGS IS DETERMINED BY OUR SENSES' LOVE OF ORDER

If now we compare the drawings that absolutely want to be seen as flat images (figures 116 and 118) with those that more or less resist a flat in-

Figures 117 and 118

The perspective representation is correct in both figures, but effective only in one and not in the other.

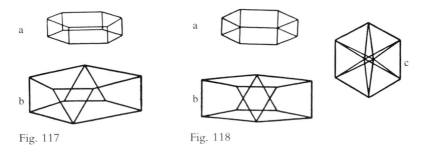

Fig. 117   Fig. 118

Figure 117

The drawing appears crooked and distorted; the three-dimensional effect is compelling, although these are not simple and ordinary solid bodies.

Figure 118

The flat interpretation is mirror symmetric, taut, and equally balanced; almost no three-dimensional effect is to be found. (c) This is the same six-sided double pyramid as figure 115.

terpretation (figures 113, 115, and 117), at first sight it becomes clear that figures 116 and 118 contain exclusively drawings of strikingly regular construction. They have at least one axis of mirror symmetry (116d, e, and f), more often there are two (116b, g, h; 118a, b, c), four (116c and i), and even six (116a and k, middle part of 118b). Many have right angles in important places (116b, c, d, g, h, i; 118a). Some contain continuous straight lines,[61] and in the effort to interpret them as solid bodies you have to split them into separate parts that are quite far removed from each other (116a and 118a) or at least kink them in depth (116c as pyramid, 116g and h; compare also figure 119), sometimes also double them either in parts or completely (116f and h; 118a). In others there are pairs of closely adjacent and, by the law of proximity,[62] tightly coupled lines, and you must again first tear them apart and put them together in wholly different directions and distances in order to obtain the solid body (116i and 118c). *Without exception these are images with good inner balance* (compare also figure 120).

61. See p. 17 section 2.

62. See p. 29 section 1.

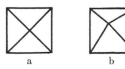

a   b

Figure 119
If the interior lines in the flat drawing are already
kinked (b), it is much easier to see a pyramid than
when the diagonal lines go straight through. Thus, in
order to represent the three-dimensional object, the
diagonals must first be bent, even though drawing (a)
is perspectively more correct than drawing (b).

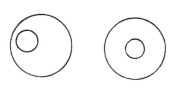

Figure 120
Two drawings that differ only in their inner balance. To see the concentric circles as a pipe or
truncated cone (lampshade) is very difficult, although you can easily imagine it. The solid form
is more easily seen with skewed circles; but here
the transition from the flat drawing to the solid-
body image is also a transition to a better balance:
the circles thereby receive a common axis, which
the concentric circles had from the beginning.

All of these regularities are missing in the seemingly three-
dimensional drawings in figures 113, 115, and 117—as long as you
perceive them as flat images. However, when interpreted as solid-body
objects, cube, roof, double pyramid, six-sided slab, and so on, they need
not shy away from competition with the flat versions of figures 116 and
118.

But this means that a flat drawing becomes three-dimensional if it
can thereby "improve" itself. Among the many possible variations of
solid-body shapes, in every case the perceptual interpretation takes on
the best possible one with the same assuredness and certainty as a freshly
formed soap bubble takes on its spherical form. For example, in figure
113b the angle between the two inclined roof surfaces could be interpreted as acute or obtuse; but you can see only a certain angle, namely,
that one with which both surfaces first act as rectangles, and second as
equally large, mirror-symmetrical rectangles. For the same reason it is
also very easy and sometimes irresistible to see a trapezoid as a diagonally
slanted square and an ellipse as a slanted circle, but difficult and almost
impossible to see a square as a slanted trapezoid and a circle as a slanted
ellipse (figure 121). You should also try this with the circles in figure 62.

It is now no longer surprising that you can turn the image of a
three-dimensional object into a flat figure without spatial meaning,
simply by providing enough inner balance for the flat percept through
suitable additions (figures 122 and 123). But there are a number of alter-

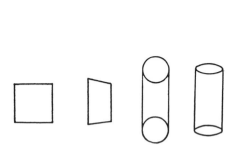

Figure 121
The two ellipses at the right look to most observers immediately like circles in inclined view, the trapezoid as an inclined square. It does not at all occur to us that the two circles on the left could also at will represent slender ellipses in more or less inclined view, and that the square could equally well be the image of an inclined trapezoid. Even if one can imagine it, it is nevertheless difficult or impossible actually to see it.

Figures 122 and 123
Disruption of the depth effect by additional features that produce a better balance in the flat drawing.

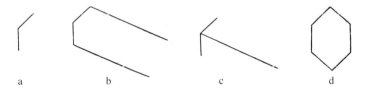

a   b   c   d

Figure 122
The inclined line in (a) can easily be seen as going into depth, like the arm of a sign-post. The same line in (c) is much more difficult, in (b) and (d) impossible to bring out of the paper's surface. In (b) and (c) the mirror symmetry of the two original lines is emphasized by the added lines; whereas in (d) the incline of the upper line is counterbalanced by opposing inclines.

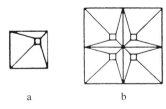

a   b

Figure 123
Whereas in (a) due to lack of balance in the flat drawing you usually perceive a truncated pyramid, in (b) after adding suitable counterweights, as a rule you only see a flat inlaid figure. Naturally for this it is a prerequisite that the eye views the entire image of (b). If you cut out part (a) from the total image by focused attention, you should not be surprised when it produces approximately the same effect in (b) as without any additions.

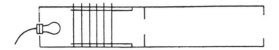

Figure 124
Set-up for depth experiments after Kopfermann (see figure 113). The wooden case is open on top for inserting the figure plates and open on the right for observation. The parallel vertical lines depict glass plates for presentation of the figure parts. The plates are actually 2 cm apart from each other. The plate farthest to the left is made of matte glass; it is lit from behind (left) and serves as a background. The interrupted line to the right of the glass plates is a cardboard pane with a round opening of about 10 cm.

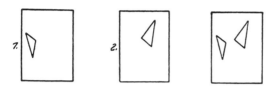

Figure 125
Two triangles on glass plates that lie behind one another (in the set-up of figure 124) that do not connect and also do not belong together are correctly seen with a depth difference of 2 cm in binocular vision as behind one another.

native and quite different interpretations that one does not think of so easily. Namely, a real three-dimensional object would have to look flat when the flat percept yields a better Gestalt than the actual one. Or for the same reason, instead of the actual spatial distribution, an equally spatial but quite different distribution should be seen. Actually, both of these can be observed to occur. If you sit (with head supported) to the right in the set-up of figure 124, and separate objects are drawn on two adjacent glass plates, as in figure 125, you can clearly see in binocular vision that they lie one behind another. But if you draw the parts of a star on three plates lying one behind another, as in figure 126, they usually merge into a real star, and even with binocular observation all the lines appear to lie in one plane. If you distribute randomly excised fragments of the drawing of a cube in a similar way onto three layers (figure 127), you do not see them in their real depth distribution either, but rather you see them as a cube. In contradiction to the laws of binocular vision you see the most regular structure that can be formed under these conditions. Naturally this no longer works when the glass plates are too far apart.

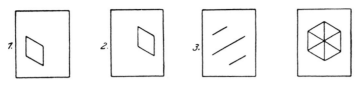

Figure 126

Pieces of figures are divided up on three glass plates lying behind one another, but so that together they form a regular coherent flat object (star) that can even be seen binocularly as a flat figure, although some of the pieces lie up to 4 cm apart. Naturally this is true only as long as one does not move back and forth.

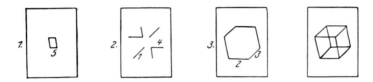

Figure 127

The individual pieces of a figure are again divided up among three plates lying behind one another. The most regular image that is possible is seen: a cube, that is, an entirely different but equally spatial arrangement in which among other things pieces 4 and 5 lie at the same distance while pieces 1 and 3 go off into depth.

In short: the law of *greatest order*, of *the good Gestalt* (prägnanz), which as we found earlier is decisive for the coherence relationships in perception, *also determines the perceived depth distribution* of geometric forms, and this often in contrast to the depth distribution that one would have to expect from the laws of binocular vision. That you can see a three-dimensional image in a drawing on the page of a book is only one—and for us an especially useful—exception to this general lawfulness.

From this point we can now finally understand how it is possible that people who have lost one eye, and even those who have seen with only one eye since birth, nevertheless find their way through space just as well as people with two eyes. Just like the latter, they see things not only next to and on top of one another, but also behind one another. Indeed, the visual space of the one-eyed person differs from that of the two-eyed only in fine details. For if the impression of depth can even occur through Gestalt forces in cases where we can see quite clearly that in reality it is only a matter of lines on a paper's surface, that should apply even more in the observation of objects in the world, where no such hindrance exists.

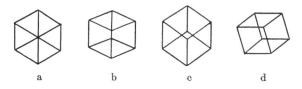

a   b   c   d

Figure 128
Four drawings of a cube. The less regular, simple, and balanced the flat drawing is, the stronger does the depth effect become. (a) Six axes of symmetry, all angles equal, three continuous straight lines that when translated into depth must be cut up in the middle and rearranged into completely different depths: no three-dimensional percept. (b) Two axes of symmetry, one continuous straight line that in part must be doubled and taken apart for the depth interpretation; only traces of a three-dimensional effect. (c) Two axes of symmetry, no continuous straight lines; noticeable depth effect. (d) No axes of symmetry, no continuous straight lines; excellent depth effect.

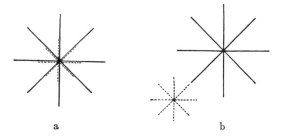

a   b

Figure 129
On the question of the depth effect through the process of enlargement. The dotted figure (solid line in the actual experiment) is presented first, the solid-line figure second. In (a) all you see is the radial rays growing longer, the depth remains apparently unchanged; whereas in (b) the entire star seems to approach in depth (see text). (From C. Calavrezo: *Über den Einfluß von Größenänderungen auf die scheinbare Tiefe. Psychol. Forschg.* 19, 1934; compare also the experiment of W. Metzger cited in figure 116.)

The law just identified has implications for the draftsman. If a line drawing is to be perceived clearly three-dimensionally, one must pay attention not only to the geometric laws of projection, but also to the psychological law of the good Gestalt. The more a flat drawing avoids regularity and tautness of structure, mirror symmetry, and inner balance in its two-dimensional configuration, the surer and more compelling the three-dimensional effect becomes (figure 128).

Even the much stronger depth effects of moving flat pictures as seen in the cinema, that can, under favorable conditions, no longer be distinguished from actual space, point under closer examination to Gestalt laws, indeed to *Gestalt laws of movement events*. To explain such laws simply and understandably, one would have to have available a movie projector instead of a printed page. But let us at least use a select example to make clear what is meant. Everyone knows the trick used in movies that an inscription, instead of simply appearing on the screen, seems to shoot toward you from a distance like an express train entering the station. Of course, in reality this is done by simply making the text grow larger. But it turns out that this effect does not work with every figure that is enlarged in this manner. It fails when the movement that transforms the small image into the larger one *is completely predetermined in the structure of the figure* and *is compatible* with it. If you project the star figure in figure 129 first as small and then, as in (a), as large *in exactly the same place* on the wall, all you see is the rays shooting outward, while the star remains stationary and at the same distance. The star appears to jump toward you as described only if you project the large image somewhat to the side, as in (b), so that the motions of the parts no longer occur along the lines of the radial rays. Suffice it to say, at this point, that as for the solid three-dimensional effects of line drawings, it is possible to formulate theoretically grounded rules also for the three-dimensional effect of ordinary movies viewed with the unaided eye.

_____

8

FORM AND SUBSTANCE OF SEEN THINGS—THE
PRÄGNANZ TENDENCY

1. A PIECE OF CLEAR WINDOW GLASS CAN LOOK OPAQUE

We are inclined to assume, without any special proof, that if an object is
transparent, its transparency would be immediately perceived. One of
the two dark strips in figure 130a is transparent—which one is it? One
looks somewhat brighter and more regular, and therefore we might assume that it is that one; but we cannot *see* it as transparent, even when
we have the actual strips in front of us instead of the figure. Well then,
we might think further, transparency may become noticeable only when
some delineated figures can be seen through the surface in question. This
is correct, but it does not explain everything. In figure 130b this requirement is fulfilled, but nevertheless no transparency is noticeable. Even
in reality it is possible to arrange those objects so that no one can see
whether the round disks lie in front of or behind the strip; for example,
if the disks are pressed firmly against the transparent strip, so that from a
distance there is no binocular depth effect.[63]

In contrast a perfectly compelling impression of transparency is
seen in figure 130c, indeed without the need for binocular vision to provide information about the depth relationships. Here the transparent
strip overlaps the letter that lies behind it: the borders of the K pass
partly inside and partly outside the overlying strip. But even that is not
what is decisive.

2. A PIECE OF GRAY CARDBOARD CAN LOOK TRANSPARENT

You can imagine figure 131b, like 131a, arising from the superposition of
a white cross and a longer black rectangle, of which one is transparent.

_____

63. Naturally in this figure no highlights should pass across the small disks, nor may
the transparent strip cast a visible deep shadow on its background. Otherwise the
depth relations are perceived the same as in figure 130c.

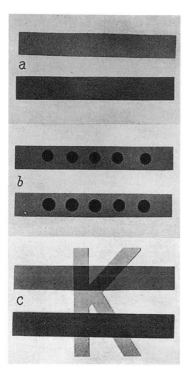

Figure 130

An experiment in transparency. (a) One of the two dark strips is transparent; which one? You can deduce it from the smoothness, but you cannot see it. (b) Even now the transparency of the upper strip is not yet clear; the round disks seem to lie on the strip instead of under it. (c) The basic requirement for apparent transparency: the strip and the letter intersect one another in such a way that each "claims as its own" the common part, since the remaining pieces alone (as in figure 27) would not be such good Gestalten. In (b) the strip appears to be uninterrupted, because it seemingly passes behind the opaque-looking disks (compare figure 3, p. 3).

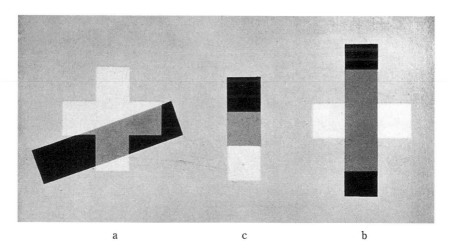

a   c   b

Figure 131

Apparent transparency. (a) Even a nontransparent piece of surface can look transparent when other bordering pieces of surface "require" it for them to form a good Gestalt. Gray paper adjacent to black and white paper then looks like the continuation of the white paper, which you see through the continuation of the (transparent)

But you cannot *see* it, even though the borders of the rectangle pass as they should, partly inside and partly outside the cross. In 131b you see a gray strip with two black rectangles at the ends, and two white rectangles on the sides, all completely opaque (the two white rectangles *could* be the ends of a continuous strip,[64] but then the gray strip does not let the least glimmer of white through). In contrast, figure 131a looks compellingly like a white cross behind a black gauze strip, or alternatively, like a black band behind a cross of milky glass—even though the occluding surface is in reality a piece of nontransparent mid-gray cardboard that was carefully glued between two white and two black pieces of cardboard. The gray paper here does not just look gray, but even when you try your best to resist it, it stubbornly appears as either black behind transparent white or white behind transparent black. If the pieces bordering the gray cardboard were rendered in color, for example, yellow and blue rather than white and black, then the plain-looking gray color would even dissolve itself into two bright opponent colors and appear yellow behind transparent blue or blue behind transparent yellow.[65]

3. ONCE AGAIN THE LAW OF THE GOOD GESTALT

But what is this strange scission of the central gray region? If you were to see the entire image in figure 131a as divided into five equally salient surfaces lying next to each other—the central gray and the remaining bordering pieces—you would have, just as in figure 27,[66] nothing but

---

64. Compare below, p. 135 section 8.

65. To portray transparent things, the artist therefore needs no transparent colors; but as we will see in a moment, must work much more carefully with opaque colors than with transparent colors.

66. Compare p. 17 section 2.

(*continued from previous page*) black strip, or, conversely, as the continuation of the black paper, which is seen through the (transparent) white one. (b) This pattern too can be seen as a black strip and a white cross—the same size as in (a)—that overlap each other. But here you clearly see three differently colored patches next to each other, with no impression of transparency. Neither the Gestalt of the black nor that of the white pieces would in any way be improved if the middle piece were added to them. (c) For the same reason as in (b), figure (c) does not separate itself into two partially overlapping rectangles but rather into three squares next to each other, even though the former is an equally valid interpretation. (Figures 130 and 131 after W. Fuchs: *Untersuchungen über das simultane Hintereinandersehen auf derselben Sehrichtung.* Z. Psychol. 91, 1923.)

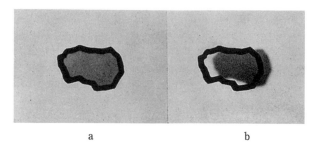

a   b

Figure 132
The spot shadow experiment of Hering. A shadow spot that exactly fills a sharply bounded bit of surface (a) looks like the color of the object. In (b) it is somewhat displaced to the side, so that it crosses the boundary line; only now does it look like a real shadow.

misshapen forms. But when the central gray piece decomposes into two layers that connect with the appropriate remaining pieces, you see nothing but well-formed objects, borders of which correspond here primarily to the law of good continuation.[67] But if as in 131c, the individual parts of the surface were so formed and assembled that the central gray patch and the remaining patches result in an organization that is just as good and simple as that of an overlapping interpretation, then transparency is no longer perceived; and transparency would even fail to appear when in reality the whole were to consist of a cross and a strip, and one of the subwholes really was transparent.[68]

When you see a bright or dark region on the surface of a body not as a colored patch, but as a spotlight or deep shadow lying transparently on the actual color, this is explained exactly the same way. A real shadow also looks exactly like a dark paint stain, and a genuine spotlight like a smooth chalk stain when it happens to exactly fill an area that is sharply delineated from its surround (figure 132a), for example, even when it completely covers a body that is floating freely in a region of different illumination. Spotlight or shadow can be identified visually only when

67. As you immediately see, in such an experiment the edges and corners of the individual pieces must abut each other very precisely; only in this way can the impression of a continuation take place. Therein too lies the difficulty for the painter that we hinted at in footnote 65.

68. The impression of transparency becomes strongest with certain shape changes of the part surfaces. In addition to the laws already mentioned, the *law of common fate* also contributes here; but this can be demonstrated only in cinema photography.

the Gestalt relations are simplified or otherwise improved by that interpretation (figure 132b).

4. A New Conception of the Law of Similarity

To the grouping principle that we learned in figure 27, a new additional
factor is seen in figure 131a: the central gray region splits not only spatially, so that instead of one layer, there are now two gray layers within
that region, but even its color is decomposed into two different tones,
each tone matching as closely as possible the tones of the adjacent white
and black regions. In the transparent perceptual interpretation therefore,
the two perceived figures, white cross and black strip, not only exhibit
the most regular spatial form, but in addition, each of them is also composed entirely of the same material: the cross is uniformly white, the
strip uniformly black. We suspect that the impression of transparency is
directly concerned with the law of similarity. With this interpretation
we have not only considerably broadened the effective range of the law
of similarity, but we have also given it a new and deeper meaning. Earlier[69] all we asserted was that regions in the visual field in which the external stimulation is similar are especially likely to form perceptual units.
But now we assert further that even regions that are joined into units for
other reasons (proximity, closure, mirror symmetry, common fate, etc.)
strive to look similar despite heterogeneous external stimulation, and
that this can, under appropriate circumstances, produce the most astonishing changes in the perceived color and material properties. Have we
not thereby attributed somewhat too much to the tendency toward similarity? We do not think so. Because again and again, even under entirely
different conditions, we can observe that regions that are immediately
adjacent exhibit a more or less uniform color in spite of the inhomoge-
neous color that might be expected on the basis of the stimulus distribution or the operation of the well-known psychological laws.

5. An Experiment on Differential Thresholds

When a disk with an interrupted stripe, as in figure 133a, is rotated
quickly, the black of the short fragments of the stripe mixes with the
white of the disk surface, resulting in the appearance of light gray rings,
as in figure 133c, which, due to the decreasing proportion of the black

---

69. See p. 32 section 3, p. 38 section 5.

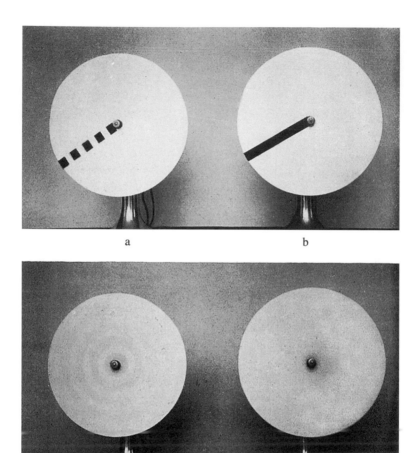

a   b

c   d

Figure 133
Color assimilation in borderless fields. With rapid rotation of disks (a) and (b) the black stripe mixes with the white of the disk. The proportion of black diminishes toward the edge, so that the mixture must become brighter there. The black stripe has the same width in both disks. Brightness would therefore have to increase in (c) and (d) toward the edge by the same degree. But only the individual separated rings on the disk with the interrupted stripe appear of different brightness (c). On the disk with an uninterrupted stripe (d), except for a very small spot around the axle, the brightness is perfectly uniform. If you touch disk (d) with the tip of a pencil halfway between the middle and the edge while it is turning, thereby producing a circular line, at the same moment the inner part of the circle becomes darker, the outer annulus brighter, while within each of those regions the brightness is again perceived to be perfectly uniform. (From K. Koffka: *Über Feldbegrenzung und Felderfüllung. Psychol. Forschg.* 4, 1923.)

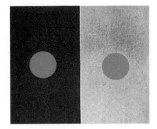

Figure 134
Brightness contrast. Basic experiment. The two round disks are cut from the same piece of gray paper. Their color looks brighter on the dark ground and darker on the white ground. If you wish to repeat this and the following experiment on a larger scale, or also with a colored ground, you should cover the entire display with a sheet of thin, unwrinkled tissue paper.

with increasing radius, become progressively lighter toward the edge, and finally invisible (subthreshold).[70] If you replace the interrupted stripe with a continuous stripe (133b), during rotation the difference in brightness with radial distance should not be less, despite the now continuous increase. Surprisingly the disk now looks equally bright from the middle to the edge (given an appropriate bandwidth) (133d). With the sharp borders of the rings eliminated, the entire surface is now so much more strongly unified that the striving for similarity becomes stronger than the stimulus difference. What is true for the entire disk is also true in figure 133c for the annular areas of the individual gray rings, especially the smallest one.

6. Some Experiments on Brightness Contrast

The bright disk in a dark surround on the left and the dark disk in a bright surround (figure 134) are in reality exactly the same shade (you can test this by laying a uniform sheet of paper with two appropriate holes over the figure). The same gray disk would look reddish if presented in a green surround, bluish in a yellow surround, and vice versa. This shift of perceived color away from adjacent contrasting colors is called *simultaneous contrast* in perceptual theory.[71] The strength of the

70. Determining the differential threshold for brightnesses was the original purpose of such disks.

71. In photography, contrast is considered to be nothing more than an abrupt difference in color or brightness.

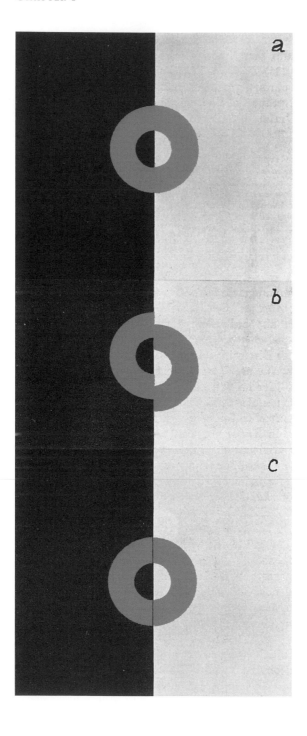

contrast depends, among other things, on the distance, chromatic saturation, and extent of the neighboring surfaces, but in addition also on the
Gestalt relationships.

Both halves of the annular ring in figure 135a should be changed
by their surround just as strongly as the two disks in figure 134. But in
fact hardly any contrast effect is noticeable. For there are not two
objects, but rather a single one (according to the laws of good continuation, of symmetry, and of closure), namely, a circular ring. Apparently
within that ring, the striving toward inner homogeneity is stronger than
the influences of the surround. If we disrupt the coherence of the circle
by cutting it into two halves with a very fine line, then the contrast is
again clearly present, even though the surround has remained exactly
the same (figure 135c).

The contrast edges that arise from the staircase-like arrangement of
three or more differently colored bands (figure 136) [in which each annular band appears darkest at its outermost perimeter although each ring
is uniformly shaded] would also be expected (on account of the decrease
of the contrast with distance) when only two differently shaded regions
border each other, or when the arrangement is not stepwise. That these
are almost never seen must also be a consequence of the striving for similarity within the individual surfaces.

In figure 135a yet another factor is in play. The unbroken circle
gives the impression of being quite independent from the surround; it
appears to lie neither in the black nor in the white region, but to lie in

◄ **Figure 135**
Contrast under various Gestalt conditions. The upper ring (a) is generally perceived
uniform gray; only occasionally does it look a shade darker on the right than on the
left. In (b) both halves are markedly different in brightness and in (c) the difference is
even stronger. In fact, all three rings have exactly the same shade: the brightness differences depend on contrast. But the more unitary the given image is configured, the
more successfully does it preserve the uniformity of its color in spite of contrast conditions. If ring (a) is separated with a stretched piece of sewing thread as in (c), then
immediately the two halves appear completely different; if you remove the thread
you see how they gradually change to resemble each other again. But as soon as
you draw the dividing line, even only in your imagination (many observers cannot
help doing this spontaneously), the difference in perceived brightness returns. If you
stretch the thread over (b), the brightness difference becomes even stronger than in
(c), for in (c) the good continuation of the annular perimeter works toward unity in
spite of the separating line. (From experiments of W. Wundt, Johann Köhler: *Arch.
Psychol.* 2, 1902; and M. Wertheimer.)

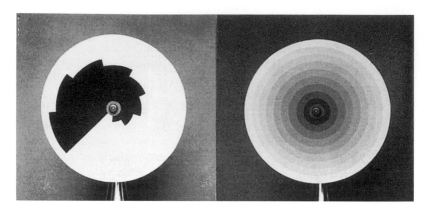

Figure 136

Edge contrast. The black ring sectors in (a), from which the rings in (b) arise during rotation, are cut off exactly radially on both ends. In reality each ring in (b) has therefore exactly the same luminance at its inner edge as at its outer one (you can convince yourself of this with the help of appropriate cover sheets). The most important cause of edge contrast is the staircase-like arrangement of the brightnesses or colors. That is why you see almost no edge contrast in the brightest ring, and none at all in the darkest ring, which lies between two equal, brighter rings. (From K. Koffka; see Figure 133.)

front of them. In the case of the cut rings in figures (b) and (c), on the other hand, the severed halves appear embedded in the black and white regions just as much as the disks in figure 134 [and thus the brightness contrast effect reappears]. A particularly strong contrast effect arises when a small colored surface that borders on other colored fields, for Gestalt reasons, is seen as a part of one of them (figure 137). For this reason the contrast effect would have to be somewhat weaker in figure 135a than in 134. But that it totally disappears for many observers is not fully explained by this alone.

7. THE GENERAL LAW OF THE GOOD GESTALT MUST ALSO BE REFORMULATED

According to the phenomena with which we have now become acquainted, the law of similarity is not just a law that selects the most homogeneous interpretation offered by the existing stimulus distribution. Rather, there are forces that under certain circumstances produce uniformity of color experience despite considerable inhomogeneity of color stimulation. If this particular conclusion were to apply not only to

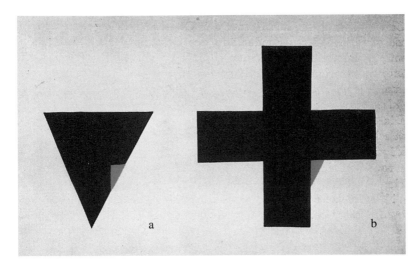

Figure 137
The significance of inclusion for contrast. (a) A black triangle, "within it" at the edge a small gray triangle. (b) Almost double the amount of black (the crosses' arms) has been added. If contrast depended only on the expanse of the surrounding surfaces, then the contrast effect of the black would have to be stronger, and thus the small gray triangle brighter. Instead it is darker than in (a), thus the effect of the black is weaker; for the small triangle now appears no longer to lie within the black figure, but next to it, within the white surround, as a result of the law of the good Gestalt, especially of good continuation and mirror symmetry. (From W. Benary: *Beobachtungen zu einem Experiment über Helligkeitskontrast. Psychol. Forschg.* 5, 1924.)

the law of similarity, but more generally to the law of the good Gestalt, then we might expect to find that a region that is merged by Gestalt forces into a unified percept—as a result of the homogeneity of its stimulus color in a differently stimulated surround—should also under the right circumstances be more regularly formed than the retinal stimulus.[72]

The depth effects discussed in the previous chapter fall under this description. The apparent purpose of these processes is to allow the perception of right-angled, mirror-symmetrical, or other regularly constructed visual objects to emerge from stimuli that on the retina have arbitrary angles or are asymmetrical, all this without even contradicting the retinal image; for the retinal image has only height and width; the depth is left indeterminate.

---

72. Compare p. 17 section 2, p. 45.

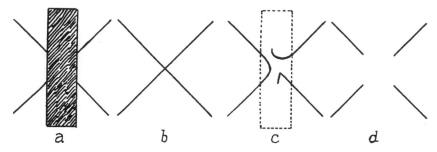

Figure 138
Overlapping. In (a) one has the immediate certainty that the diagonal lines continue under the shaded rectangle, and indeed that they cross, as in (b). When it turns out with removal of the rectangle that the lines continue quite differently (c) or even that they stop right at the edge of the rectangle (d), one feels deceived; the impression of a straight continuation was that compelling.

8.   OVERLAPPING

The perceptual tendency toward the good Gestalt, though, has even broader implications. What do you see in figure 138a? Two intersecting lines, as in figure 138b, except with the point of intersection occluded. For the observer this is more than just an abstract conjecture; the impression is self-evident and compelling.[73] So much so that you would feel outright deceived if, on removal of the covering strip, it turned out that the lines were configured something like in figure 138c or did not intersect at all (138d). You can try this experiment on someone with an actual occluding strip, and watch the expression on his face when exposing picture (c). It seems clear therefore that in (a) the occluded parts of the cross behaved exactly as if you could actually see them; they were

---

73. This is the reason why, without thorough practice, it is also an almost insoluble task for an unprejudiced and conscientious person (for example, in court) to separate in his observations what certainly was perceived from what was only suspected. For much of what the prosecuting judge—from his point of view rightly so—calls sheer speculation belongs to the large domain of that which (like the crossing of the lines in figure 138a) completes itself so compellingly and entirely without our having anything to do with it, that nothing at all remains for the observer to conjecture about, i.e., to deliberate and complete in thought. Hence too the confusion of the inexperienced witness and the feeling of losing his footing when it is demonstrated to him indisputably that after all he had reported only a conjecture.

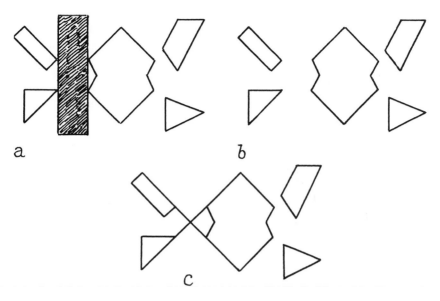

Figure 139
Figure (a) contains on both sides of the gray rectangle the same four diagonal lines as 138a. But here the lines do not have the slightest tendency to continue underneath the rectangle. If you remove the rectangle (b) it is self-evident that its place is empty. The continuation and connection of the four lines would not simplify or otherwise make the image better, but would only make it more confused (c).

invisibly present. [Translators' note: Michotte et al. (1991) have since named this type of invisible percept *amodal* completion, because the experienced structure is not expressed in any particular sensory modality, such as color, brightness, texture, or motion.*]

But it can also be different. In figure 139a you would be particularly astonished if the corresponding four diagonal lines were connected as in figure 139c. Although geometrically they continue exactly as in figure 138, here they do not have the slightest tendency to link up and complete themselves under the occluding strip, because they are already

---

* Michotte, A., Thinès, G., & Crabbe, G. (1991). Amodal Completion of Perceptual Structures. In G. Thinès, A. Costall, & G. Butterworth (Eds.), *Michotte's Experimental Phenomenology of Perception* (pp. 140–167). Hillsdale, NJ: Lawrence Erlbaum Associates. (Original work published in 1967.)

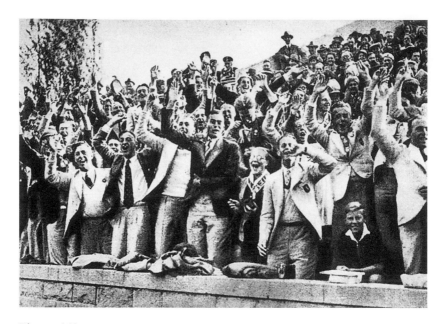

Figure 140
The effect of the *invisibly present* in perception: look at a crowd of people. Of all the people you see none completely, of most of them only a fragment of a face or arm. Nevertheless in no way do you have the impression of standing in front of a collection of arms and more or less complete heads, etc. (Photo from *Hör mit mir*, Schacht-Verlag, Bochum.)

organized externally into simple Gestalten (figure 139b). In this case, adding the lines under the strip would make the picture anything but simpler or improved. Something totally strange would be added, something not at all implied in the image. So again, the invisibly present crossing seen in figure 138a is a special case of perceptual striving toward a good Gestalt. Indeed, you can confirm this for yourself with every glance around your environment, for example, when viewing a crowd of people (figure 140), a case of greatest importance in everyday life.

Moreover, this example is one of the cases in which acquired knowledge plays a role together with Gestalt laws. Knowledge becomes ever more decisive a factor the less simple the structure of the image that requires completion, and thus the greater the probability that the occluded portion has characteristics that are not strictly determined by the visible parts of the stimulus. Nevertheless, the impression that the

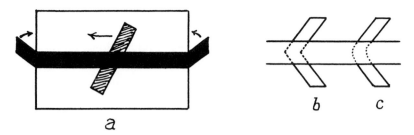

Figure 141
Another example of apparent transparency. The (nontransparent) black strip in (a) is
fastened with its folded-over ends on a white card (real size for best effect is 3–4 times
larger than depicted). As long as you move the colored strip (hatched in the drawing)
back and forth behind it, you get the distinct impression under subdued lighting of
seeing its color right through the black band. If the colored strip has a corner, as in
(b), the portion shining through looks bent, as in (c). Aside from the knowledge of
specifically this piece of paper, however, there is no general experience to which this
effect could be attributed. (From O. Rosenbach: *Z. Psychol.* 29, 1902.)

occluded figure does not terminate abruptly at the occluding edge, but
continues on behind it is even in these cases independent of our knowledge of the partially occluded objects.

Just as with the depth effect of line drawings, as a rule the retinal
image is adhered to in the completion of the occluded portion; the missing pieces therein are indeed "as good as there" perceptually; literally
they are as effective as if they were actually seen, but they nevertheless
remain invisible. But here it sometimes happens that the retinal evidence
is simply overridden. You can fasten a strip of opaque black paper across
the front of a piece of white cardboard, folding the ends of the strip behind the card (figure 141). If you now slide a bright colored strip, for
example yellow, between the card and the black strip, back and forth
with irregular movements, then, especially under somewhat subdued illumination, the invisible completion becomes visible. You believe you
can see the yellow color quite clearly through the black strip. This experiment demonstrates particularly clearly the distinction between immediate Gestalt effects and the effects of knowledge and experience,
and also of behavior. For example, if you fold the colored strip to form
a sharp corner and slide it so that the corner remains occluded, the com-
pleted piece is seen as curved instead of angular (figures 141b and c) despite your better knowledge; the perceived shape does not care about
our knowledge and our expectation.

9. THE EFFECT OF UNFAVORABLE VIEWING CONDITIONS

There are also conditions of the most diverse kinds—similar to those in the threshold and contrast experiments above—under which the greater regularity of the perceived form is achieved in apparent contradiction to the retinal image.

When certain errors occur under unfavorable viewing conditions, inasmuch as the perceived shapes deviate to a greater or lesser degree from the actual shapes, nobody is surprised, just as when in target shooting the bullet holes deviate more frequently and farther from the center of the target, the more unfavorable the shooting conditions. If the deviations were purely due to chance, then (when averaged over enough trials) they would be distributed uniformly in all directions. Similarly, if perceptual errors were due purely to chance, then one would expect that a regular shape should look irregular just as often as an irregular one looks regular; and second, that with a slightly irregular shape, an appearance that is too regular should occur only as one among many other, in part much too irregular appearances. In reality, in such observations the errors are not distributed randomly, but are surprisingly uniformly distributed. Among a hundred shapes that look more regular than they really are, there is maybe one for which the opposite is the case. Whatever the particular type of observation difficulty, whether the presented images are too small and distant (figure 142), are too faint and blurred (figure 143), or lie too far in peripheral vision (figure 144), or whether they are tactile images felt with eyes closed (figure 145; compare also figure 55c[74]) is irrelevant. Virtually without exception the mistake in the perceived image is that it is structured more unitarily, more tightly, and more regularly than the stimulus pattern even where the articulation remains quite intact.[75] The perceptual image generally is not actually wrong, but rather to the contrary, it seems to define a basic form or skeleton, a more perfect original image, from which the real object only seems to be diverted through certain distortions, deletions or additions.

The striving for similarity may therefore be subsumed under a general striving toward order and unity (the prägnanz tendency), the effective domain of which far transcends the mere selection of the most favorable segmentation of the perceptual field.[76]

---

74. See p. 44 section 1

75. Compare p. 50ff section 3, p. 56 section 5.

76. See p. 8 section 6, p. 17 section 2, and p. 29 section 1.

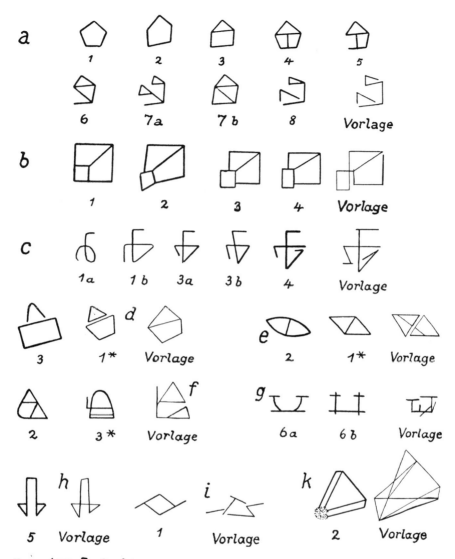

* andere Beobachter

Figure 142

Unfavorable observation conditions 1: smallest Gestalten. Presented patterns (in reality white lines on a black ground) are observed through a concave reducing glass and are enlarged step by step from approximately the size of a dot. Numbers indicate size steps, 1 the smallest, 8 the largest; the last figure in each series depicts the stimulus pattern itself [labeled Vorlage; * different observers]. **(a)** Complete development of a figure through all 8 steps for one subject: initial figure closed, without filling of the interior, regular polygon (1), then transition to a structure composed of a square and (*continued from previous page*) triangle (2, 3), inner lines initially parallel and at right angles to the outer lines (4, 5); with 7b still a reversion to a closed outer perimeter. **(b) and (c)** Some characteristic stages from the development of other figures in the same subject. (b) At first a square enclosure, in which there is a second square and a connecting line that runs along a mirror axis; in the emergence of the small rectangle (1b) temporary unification on the basis of the oblique, thereafter again large square and small rectangle on top of it. (c) At first a nearly regularly curved loop (1a), but immediately formation of the most important partial stretches (1b), the left end stretches parallel and equally long with the lower half of the main vertical; in 3b temporary orientation of the main straight line toward the left end stretches; the first indication of the inner line on the right (4) parallel to the main horizontal. **(d–k)** A number of individual shapes of different figures and subjects. (d) Variation toward a rectangle and isosceles or even equilateral triangle. (e) Smoothing and simplification toward a lens or rhomboid; only the favorably positioned inner line is, although simplified, seen from the beginning. (f) Closure, mirror symmetry, smoothing of the edge line, omission of the "appendix"; orientation of inner lines parallel to outer lines (2) and to each other (3). (g) Both drawings are mirror-symmetrical and also otherwise uniform: all horizontals stand out (6a), all lines are crossed (6b). (h) Drawing mirror-symmetrical; stem lines vertical and parallel, upper closing horizontal, lower triangles mirror identical. (i) Drawing: rhomboid lying horizontally, with two sides extended. (k) Drawing mirror-symmetrical, inner lines parallel to the outer edges. (From E. Wohlfahrt: *Der Auffassungsvorgang an kleinen Gestalten. N. Psychol. Stud.* 4, 1932.)

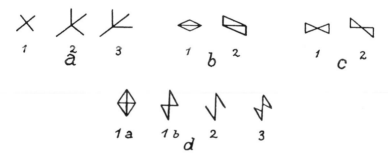

Figure 143
Unfavorable observation conditions 2: low-contrast stimuli. The images emerge in moderate size very gradually from their background as the contrast is gradually increased. Here, for example, instead of the three-pronged fork [stimulus pattern] you see at first a simple oblique cross (a); instead of the oblique parallelogram a straight level rhomboid (b), instead of the likewise oblique figure c_2 the form of a horizontal hourglass. The hooklike object d_3 looks in 1a completely closed and mirror-symmetrical, in 1b at least both the small diagonal lines are fused with the rectangular continuous connecting line (interpretations 1a and 1b come from different observers). (From K. Gottschaldt: *Über den Einfluß der Erfahrung auf die Wahrnehmung von Figuren II. Psychol. Forschg.* 12, 1929).

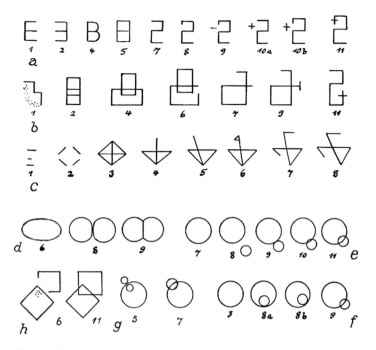

Figure 144

Unfavorable observation conditions 3: observation in peripheral vision. The figures always appear for a short duration in a moderate size with strong contrast, but at first far in the visual periphery, then stepwise increasingly closer. At 1 the deviation amounts to about 90°, at 11 it is 0°, i.e., the figure lies exactly in the line of sight. **(a)** After there was initially the vague impression of something like a horizontally divided Latin letter, in 5 for the first time there appears a closed, mirror-symmetrical initial figure, from which in 7 the no longer mirror-symmetrical skeleton emerges through deletion of parts of the enclosure. The small cross seems inconsistent with the rest of the figure; it therefore only makes sense that (in 10a) it also at first seems to be spatially segregated; compare also (e) and (f). **(b)** First unclear fragments, then at once a closed initial figure (2), which dissolves into two closed partial figures (4), everything mirror-symmetrical. With this observation the perception of intersections plays a role quite early (already in 4), whereas even after the transition to a single [self-crossing] line (7) the direction of the bend remains the same to the end. **(c)** Here too the perceived pattern, as soon as it becomes clear (2, 3), is closed, right-angled, multiply mirror-symmetrical. In this experiment you can see particularly clearly how there is a step-by-step departure from this highest degree of order until finally the stimulus pattern is attained (the real mirror axis of the presented pattern plays psychologically no role because of its unfavorable orientation). **(d)** Not only the horizontal ellipse (6), but according to the one-sidedness of contour lines (chapter 1 section 5, figure 11) also the pair of closed rings (8) is psychologically simpler than the presented stimulus pattern (9). **(e–h)** Overlapping intersection of independent features is psychologically a difficult and late-emerging property (compare p. 44ff.). Under unfavorable observation conditions there are various remedies: often one of the figures is simply suppressed entirely (e_7 and f_3) or partially (h_6); or it gets cut apart (g_5); or the small figure moves into the large one (f_8); or both figures pull completely apart (e_8). Displacement as a remedy has been observed so far only in peripheral vision. (From an unpublished study in the Psychol. Institut, Frankfurt am Main)

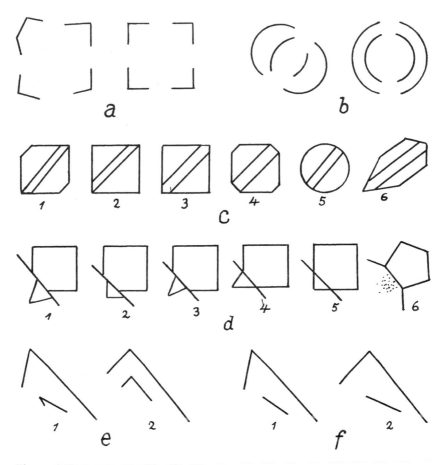

Figure 145
Unfavorable observation conditions 4: tactile Gestalten. The figures are embroidered
on cards and are felt with eyes closed. In this figure the presented pattern is always
on the left, to the right next to it is a sample of shapes as they were drawn by different observers after feeling the stimulus. **(a)** Almost without exception the square form
is produced. **(b)** Mostly the bent arc pieces are arranged around a vertical mirror axis.
In addition, the size of the two inner ones becomes balanced, and very often they
appear as parts of two concentric circles. **(c)** Usually production of the square shape
and of the precisely diagonal course of the inner lines (2, 3), in 3 furthermore there
is a mirror-symmetrical arrangement into an exactly diagonal band. Or alternatively,
rounding-off of all corners (4) all the way to complete rounding (5). In a third kind
of unification (6) everything conforms to the oblique (as in figure 142b$_2$). **(d)** The
warped and noncollinear section on the lower left becomes among other things
right-angled and parallel to the sides of the square (2), or in an orderly way is shifted
to the middle (3), and attached to the sides of the square as a continuation (4); finally
it serves exclusively as the completion of the square. In 6, the relationships on the

(*continued from previous page*) lower left are still unclear; here the cut-off square is presented as a pentagon with appendices, and at the same time it is strongly modified in the direction of a regular pentagon. **(e)** The two hooks (1) are usually positioned parallel and often also both equidistant from the corners (2). **(f)** If the short end is omitted from the smaller hook in (e), the remaining line rotates exactly in the opposite direction. Now the whole triangle emerges, and the lower line assumes the direction of the baseline. It should be noted that in all experiments the observers had no idea of their enhancement of the stimulus, but rather presumed that they had reproduced the figures quite veridically. (From an unpublished study of J. Becker.)

9

Gestalt Laws in the Spatial Effects of Brightness

As we found in chapter 7, the depth effect of perspective drawings is best understood through the law of the good Gestalt. We would now like to see whether the discovery that we made there with line drawings also helps us to understand the spatial effects of light and shadow.

1. A Depth Effect of the Matching of Brightness Distributions

Even if you actually stand in front of the wall in figure 146 (at a distance of 4–6 m), you believe that you are seeing a rectangular hole to the right, behind which at some distance there is a farther wall with patterned wallpaper. But on the left it looks like a piece of wallpaper that has been affixed to the nearer wall as long as you stand perfectly still. Only when you move back and forth, or come so close that the depth effect of binocular vision becomes predominant, do you notice that the left wallpaper is also located on a farther wall seen through a rectangular aperture, like the one on the right. But even when you stand quite close, the tendency of the left stimulus to pull itself into the front wall is still clearly noticeable; as long as you stand still, you have the impression that the left wall is not as far behind the near wall as the right one, even when the distance is actually exactly the same (in this experiment both were 1 m behind the front wall). But why? Because the brightness distribution on the left piece of wallpaper is so consistent with the distribution of light on the front wall, as if it were a part of it. This consistency of the brightness distributions on the rear and the front walls thus has exactly the same effect as the consistency of the single pieces of the star that lie behind each other in figure 126.

2. The Law of Similarity

The left piece of wallpaper not only looks spatially closer, but furthermore it appears considerably more uniform than the right one. You

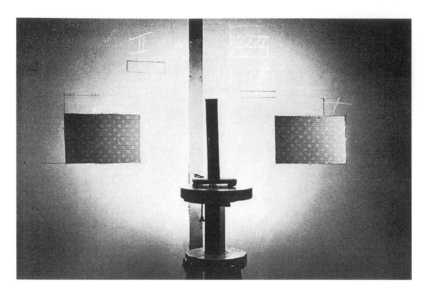

Figure 146
Depth effect of the brightness distribution. A wall illuminated from the center; left
and right, rectangular apertures, and 1 m back beyond it a second wall with striped
wallpaper. But only on the right where the brightness gradient on the back wall is
different from that on the front wall do you see that it is farther away. On the left,
by contrast, where the brightness gradients are consistent, the wallpaper seems to be
glued to the near wall. (From M. Turhan: *Über eine räumliche Wirkung von Helligkeits-
gefällen. Psychol. Forschg.* 21, 1935.)

really get the impression of a colored paper with approximately equal
reflectance, which is only perceived to be somewhat closer to the light
at its right edge. This impression is not in the least disturbed when the
brightness gradient is painted on the rear piece of paper, so that in reality
it is not caused by the illumination, even when the observer knows
about it. Sometimes, especially when you close one eye, you can see—
even in reality—the right piece of wallpaper also on the near wall, or
even somewhat closer than the near wall. But in this case it never looks
flat, but always as though it were fastened to the wall at the center with
two thumbtacks on top and bottom, but at both sides bent toward you
in an arc. And in this case the right field also appears to be of uniform
reflectance, but only under nonuniform *illumination*.

We want to follow this track further. If you manage to see the
convex-folded card in the middle of figure 147, which is lit from the
left, as a flat, irregular six-sided surface, or even as folded backward (con-

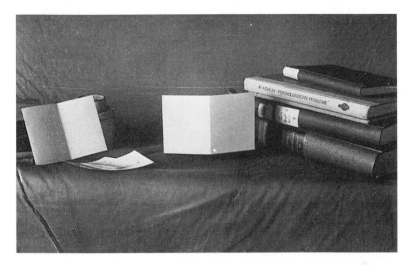

Figure 147
The bent card. Look at the convex fold of the card at the center. The card appears—in reality even more clearly than in the figure—uniformly white, but merely more brightly illuminated on the left panel. But if you succeed in seeing the card with a concave fold (open to the front) so that the dark panel seems to lie in the light and the bright panel in the shadow, the card also no longer looks uniformly colored, but rather radiantly bright on the left and pitch black on the right. Only the first, in this case correct, spatial interpretation conforms to the law of similarity; and therefore this configuration is seen much more easily than the second.

cave) and opening out toward the observer, then, aside from the rectangular form of both halves, the homogeneity of the color is also immediately lost. If you see it as a flat surface, it appears to consist of one white and one dark gray-colored panel. If you see it folded concave, then the right panel, now apparently turned toward the light, becomes pitch black, but the left panel, apparently turned away from the light, becomes so brilliant that it is easy to believe that it has become translucent and light is penetrating through it from the back. In the correct spatial interpretation, however, when the fold is seen as convex, the card appears uniformly white despite the brightness difference of the two panels, with the left panel turned toward the light and the right panel away from the light. This appears even more vivid in reality than in the picture. If this spatial interpretation is much easier to see than either the flat one or the one bent the other way, we see again a familiar law of organization at work that we already know: the law of similarity. In this specific case the law would read: *All parts of the surface of an apparently coherent structure tend toward that spatial configuration in which the intrinsic color of the perceived object becomes as uniform as possible, so that all extant differences in brightness can be attributed to mere differences in illumination.* As the three-dimensional effect of shadowed pictures demonstrates, this tendency is independent of whether the brightness differences are actually differences in illumination of a real body, or only differences in the coloration [or reflectance] of a surface that is actually flat.

According to the effects that the tendency toward uniformity of coherent figural surfaces may have on the apparent material nature (transparency) and also on contrast and threshold phenomena, it is no longer too bold to assume that this tendency is also able to decisively influence the perceived spatial arrangement and orientation of colored surfaces.

3. Application to the Portrayal of Volumetric Forms

Some illustrations of relief pictures, whether you want them to or not, look inverted in depth in the sense that all hills look like valleys, and all valleys like hills. Many of them most stubbornly resist all efforts to turn them right side up again in depth.

Yet for the most part one can restore them fairly easily by turning the book upside down or sideways, and then taking another look (figure 148). What happens when, for example, the picture is turned upside down? The light and dark edges in the picture have changed places; if the bright edges had been below and to the right, they are now above and to the left. In reading and looking at pictures, objects that exhibit highlights from the top or left generally appear preferably as elevations (mountains, mounds, ridges) whereas those with highlights from below and to the right appear as depressions (valleys, channels, tracks, impressions). But why? When we read under ideal illumination, the light comes from the top left. Therefore in this illumination the depicted surfaces appear correctly as uniformly colored only when highlights appear on the upper left, and contrariwise shadows to the lower right (see also figure 149).

Thus if you wish to avoid the undesirable inversion of relief photos, you must be careful that when you take the picture, the light falls on the object from exactly the same direction as the light that will later illuminate the page when the book is being read, that is, from the upper left.

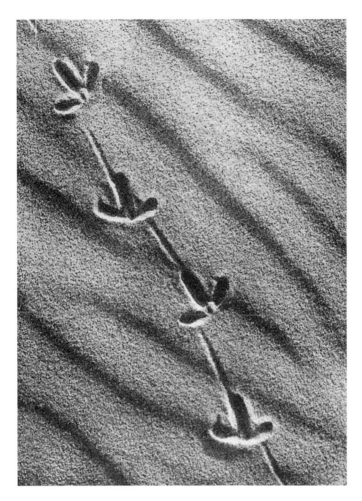

Figure 148
A not entirely unambiguous relief photo; you sometimes see ridges instead of grooves. The lighting in such a photo, like the light from a properly positioned reading lamp, must come from above left. To achieve this, turn the book counter-clockwise with the left edge of the picture toward the bottom, and then the tracks become unambiguous grooves. If you turn the book clockwise, with the right edge toward the bottom, you can see almost only the ridges; these too then appear to be lit from the upper left. (Tracks of the grey plover in dune sand, $^1/_3$ natural size; figure from *Natur und Volk* 63, p. 379, 1933.)

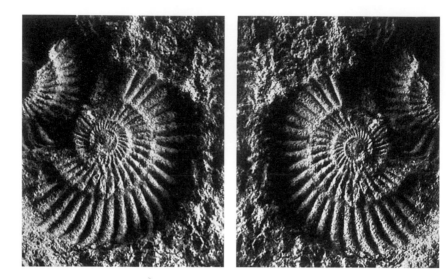

Figure 149

The same photo presented twice, of the impression of an ammonite (*Parkinsonia* sp., Middle Jurassic), on the right, printed correctly, on the left, printed reversed left to right. Thus the photographer has intentionally achieved the objective that the photo on the left looks like the [convex] fossil that made the [concave] impression on the right. The effect is especially compelling if you turn the page clockwise with the right edge toward the bottom. (Photo Hut, Basel [Leica]; graciously supplied by Priv.-Doz. Dr. Rittmann, Basel.)

If the photographer (or the printer) failed to follow this rule, or was prevented due to external factors, the reader can usually compensate by turning the book until the light in the picture has the same direction as the reading light. In figure 148, for example, the track is seen correctly when the bright highlights appear to the lower right.

The perceptual preference for illumination from the upper left is even observed (although somewhat less so) when the picture happens to be viewed under reverse illumination, that is, with light coming from the lower right. Thus when reading, our eye, not us, for we are normally quite naive in this, "expects" the light to come from the upper left, even when it is actually oriented differently. This is undoubtedly a consequence of experience, namely, habituation to the most common direction of illumination. But it is easy to verify that depth impression becomes more vivid and stable when you hold the book somewhat at a distance while at the same turning, so that the direction of illumination is now consistent with that of the photograph.

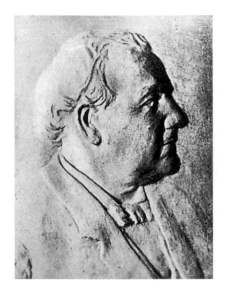 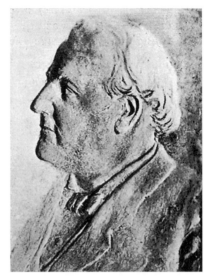

Figure 150
It is impossible to perceive hollow reliefs of human faces correctly; faces can appear
only as convex solid volumes, even though this makes the lighting quite unlikely and
inverted from the lower right, or even as black light from above left. To the left the
convex solid form, to the right the concave hollow form, both lit from above left.
(Figures 150 and 152 from Luckiesh: *Light and Shade and Their Applications*. New
York, 1916.)

4. THE LAWS OF PROXIMITY AND CLOSURE

Certain examples of relief photos contradict the perceptual tendency
outlined above. For example, photographs of hollow reliefs of human
faces appear exclusively as solid convex shapes, preferring to create their
own completely unnatural direction of illumination that is contradictory
to the prevailing illumination at the moment (figure 150).

In the case of faces, undoubtedly familiarity plays a role. But this is
not quite so certain in the case of ripples left in sand by flowing water
(figure 151). In spite of the almost precisely correct lighting (see the
shadow on the pocket watch), the ripples stubbornly appear to some
observers as some sort of ridges that are lit from the right; such ridges
are not exactly something you see every day. But the influence of familiarity becomes quite improbable when in figure 152 the left image, instead of appearing as a hemispherical hollow, is seen as a sphere, just as
the right one, and furthermore with the very unlikely illumination from

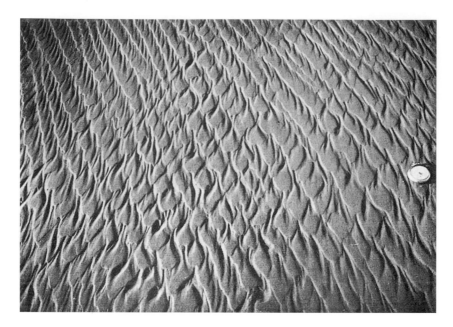

Figure 151

In the photograph of this natural relief pattern—tracks made by flowing water on a beach—the illumination was almost exactly correct; as the shadow and highlight on the watch show, it came from the left. Nevertheless many observers see only ridges rather than furrows. If you do not see the picture correctly from the outset, just focus on the narrow area around the watch's shadow [or turn the picture by 180 degrees]; instead of narrow streaks you should thereby try to see (approximately drop-shaped) smooth spots as figure or pattern, for the pattern strives to stand out spatially. (From *Natur und Volk* 65, p. 521, 1935.)

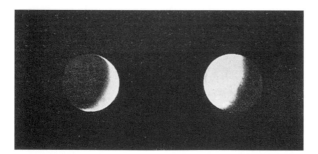

Figure 152

Spatial emergence of the figure in the simplest arrangement. You see two spheres with opposite illumination; in reality both objects are illuminated from the same direction, and the left one is a hollow hemisphere.

the right rear. At least observers who have been drinking their coffee and tea for years from approximately hemispherical concave cups, and particularly those who work daily with pots and bowls, should be sufficiently familiar with hemispherical hollows of this type. It also goes against all experience in figure 97 when the groove left by a pencil looks not like a groove but like a ridge (which moreover is lit from the right). This is how a page with mirror writing would appear on the reverse side of a page, which is something that barely one person in a thousand has ever seen in a lifetime.

But we already know a very similar phenomenon: in flat drawings, small and enclosed surface patches tend as a rule to assume the status of figure, that is, as solid filled-in objects, and the larger surrounding surfaces as ground, as empty space before which the figure appears.[77] The impression of an empty space in an otherwise stable and continuous environment (for example, a hole in a plank) is much less common among simple surface figures and usually does not arise there by itself. If we assume that the laws of closure and proximity are also operative for the perception of depth relationships among solid volumetric bodies, the results would be exactly what we found in figures 150–152 and 97. The interior surface of spatially curved surface patches would preferentially appear solid and filled-in, the outside as empty surround, and the tighter the curvature of the perimeter of the patch, the stronger the effect; that is, small surface patches should tend to appear as solid figural forms, and only with great difficulty would they appear as depressions or voids.

5. THE LAW OF SYMMETRY

In figure 149 (and also in figure 150) yet another Gestalt law that we have discussed becomes apparent. Although the direction of illumination in figure 149 is just right, some observers see the right-hand picture as a convex body. In order to see it as hollow, they have to rotate the page clockwise, with the right edge downward, even though in doing so the illumination appears to come from the right, and is therefore less favorable than in the upright orientation. This appears to be related to the fact that both pictures are arranged symmetrically; for the described effect becomes more compelling the more one permits the pair of pictures to act as a mirror-symmetrical total unit. The symmetry of the

---

77. See p. 10ff.

two halves is, however, complete only when the depth relationships on both sides match, that is, when both pictures are seen either as convex or both as hollow. Apparently for some observers, symmetry in the visual field exerts so strong an influence that it prevails even at the cost of a globally consistent pattern of illumination. The fact that both sides are generally seen as convex solids, but almost never as hollow voids, depends of course on the law of closure. That the influence of symmetry decreases strongly as soon as the pictures are presented vertically, rather than horizontally adjacent, is not surprising. In general, symmetry about a vertical axis is perceived much more readily and saliently than that about a horizontal axis. Only left and right are completely equivalent to each other as spatial regions; for above and below this is not the case.

6. OVERVIEW

In the course of our preliminary test of the regularities in the depth effect of brightness we met more old acquaintances than we dared hope for in the beginning: from the spatial conglomerative effect of fitting together, due to the (here more basic) law of similarity and the laws of proximity and closure to the law of symmetry. Up to this point these phenomena have been presented as a preliminary collection of individual examples. But verification through systematically performed experiments is under way, and we can look forward with confidence to their eventual results.

10
———

YET ANOTHER IMPORTANT CAMOUFLAGE PRINCIPLE

1. CASES IN WHICH COLOR ADAPTATION ALONE IS INSUFFICIENT

The speckled hen in figure 153 stands in front of a wall that is covered all over with the same feathers that the chicken itself bears. After all that has been said earlier about camouflage, we would have to expect that with such perfect correspondence of color and pattern, the shape of the animal would disappear into its surroundings. But that is not at all the case; in comparison with almost all the different cases discussed earlier, the camouflage here fails spectacularly. The same is true for the grouse in figure 154. It is exactly the same white color as the snow, but its camouflage is frankly deplorable. It stands out even more sharply, more saliently, and, for a hungry predator, more invitingly against an environment of the same color, than the white alpine hare in figure 155 against the nearly black background at the edge of the forest.

2. THE CURVATURE OF THE BODY IS THE BETRAYER, LIGHT AND SHADOW ARE ITS ACCOMPLICES

What is lacking here becomes clear when we look once again at the picture of a woodcock (figure 156), the same kind of bird that was so superbly camouflaged in figure 71. Here you see the animal at first glance, even if not quite as clearly as the birds in figures 153 and 154. But why is the camouflage now so imperfect? True, the environment is indeed not exactly the same as in figure 71, and the position of the bird is also a bit different, because this time it is not a living bird; but none of this is crucial. What is decisive is the visible roundness of the body. This rotundity, which is so characteristic of the body form of most animals, must still be removed for the eye of the beholder. Only then can the principles of camouflage described earlier come to full effect.[78] Those

---

78. The only exception is camouflage according to the law of belongingness, when the body of the animal is supposed to become one of many things in the surrounding, which themselves possess a similar volumetric rotundity (pebbles, bits of twigs, etc.).

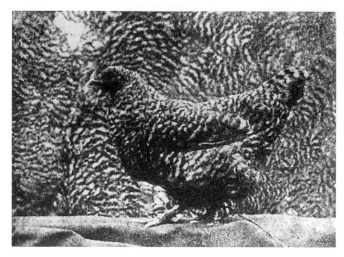

Figure 153
Speckled hen (Plymouth rock breed) in front of a wall that is covered with skins of the same kind of chicken. The animal is clearly visible, despite its perfect homogeneity with the environment. (Figures 152 and 153 from Thayer: *Concealing Coloration in the Animal Kingdom*. New York, 1902.)

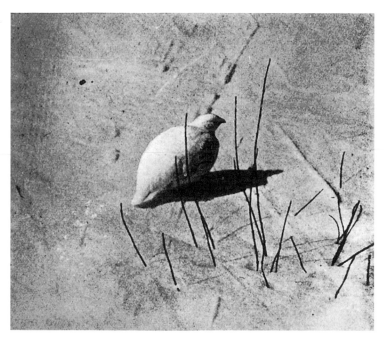

Figure 154
The North American grouse is, despite its snow-white winter plumage, poorly camouflaged. It stands out unmistakably from its environment.

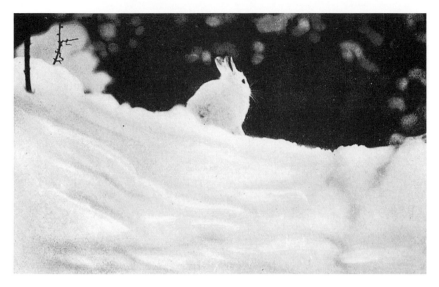

Figure 155
Alpine hare in the most unfavorable position (like figs. 87–89): white in front of the
dark forest edge, but still not as visible as the grouse in figure 154. (Figure 155 from
Natur und Museum 59, p. 268, 1929.)

principles are thus almost without exception sufficient only for flat
objects, such as flounders, butterfly wings, and the like.

But why does the roundness of the body strike the eye so strongly
in figure 156, and by contrast not at all in figure 71? For binocular vision
it is no different, and not only in the picture where everything is flat, but
also in reality, where both bodies have rounded features. But we already
know now that the bodily roundness of seen objects can be due to
something entirely different than binocular cues. The crucial factor is
that for the woodcock in figure 156, as for the grouse in the sun, there
is a substantial brightness difference between back and belly that was
completely absent in the bird in figure 71 and for the alpine hare at the
edge of the forest. This is the same phenomenon as in the sphere in figure 105, which looks really like a sphere only when illuminated from
one direction, but is indistinguishable from a flat disk in completely diffuse illumination.

But whereas in the case of the hare its invisibility is due to fortunate weather conditions, with completely diffuse illumination shining as
strongly from below as from above on a gray winter day, in the case of
the woodcock it is due to the brightness profile across its plumage.

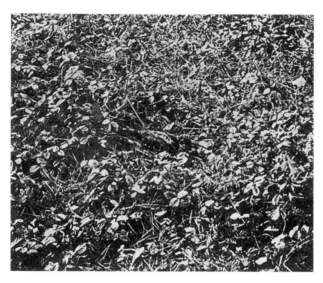

Figure 156
Woodcock (dead specimen) in similar position and environment as in figure 71, but here clearly visible, because the underside was artificially colored to the same darkness as the back. (Figures 156–158 from Thayer; see figure 153.)

3.   COUNTERSHADING AS THE SOLUTION

How would the body of an animal living outdoors, under the light of the sky and the sun, have to be colored to appear uniformly bright from top to bottom, and thus to lose its bodily roundness for the eye? You would have to color the most brightly lit parts of its coat dark, and color those parts lying in the deepest shadow bright, if possible in such a way that differences in illumination and in coloration precisely cancel each other (figure 157). This countershading is absent on the woodcock in figure 156. Its belly is colored brown, the same color as its back; as a result the brightness difference stands out, and with it the roundedness of the body, and therefore the animal is plainly visible. Now we understand why so many animals—aside from their normal camouflage coloring and markings—have a dark back and a light belly (figure 158). However, not all animals have this simple brightness distribution. With caterpillars and pupae of many types of butterflies countershading occurs twice: first at the place that is turned toward the light, and again on both sides (figure 159). The result is that the volumetric shape of the animal does not only disappear under appropriate illumination, but furthermore

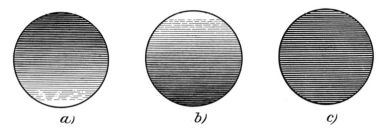

a) b) c)

Figure 157
Thayer's law, according to which countless animal species are protected from the volumetric effect of light and shadow. The animals are shaded as in (a), the sky illuminates them as in (b), and the two effects cancel each other as in (c). The distribution of light and shadow, through which non-transparent bodies become recognizable as such for the eye, is thus completely obliterated. (Thayer, p. 14.)

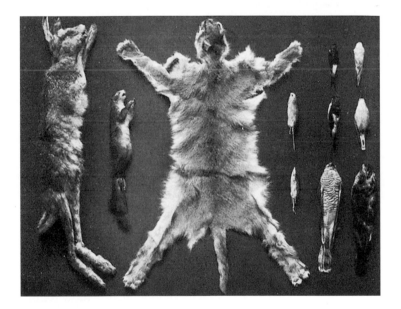

Figure 158
Animal and bird skins with countershading camouflage. From left to right and from above to below: field hare, squirrel, desert lynx, field mouse, water shrew, two house martin swallows, two red-headed shrikes, two sparrow hawks. (From the collections of the Natur-Museum Senckenberg, Frankfurt am Main)

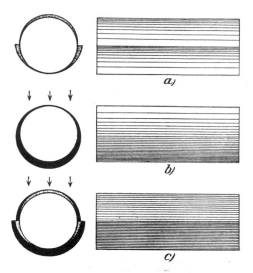

Figure 159
The most common type of countershading in caterpillars and pupae
of butterflies. Left, cross section
of the animal; right, the view
from the side. (a) Distribution of
color: countershading occurs twice.
(b) Distribution of the light. (c)
The result of the combined effect
of (a) and (b): two monotone,
thus flat-appearing bands of different brightness. (Figures 159–161
from F. Süffert: *Phänomene visueller Anpassung* I–III. *Z. Morph.
Ök. Tiere.* 26, 1932.)

it fractures into two separate part surfaces that under the right conditions
appear like a partially folded leaf (figures 160 and 161).

Even the direction of shading is not always the same in all animals.
The shading from dark to light does not always go from the back to the
belly. That is useful only for animals that usually turn their belly toward
the earth and their back toward the sky, especially while resting. Animals
with different resting postures also need a different direction of shading,
whether from belly to back, or from head to tail, and so on. It even happens that the same animal during the course of its development assumes
opposite shadings. The caterpillar of the Clouded Yellow butterfly (*Colias edusa*) sits mostly with its back toward the light (see figure 166), the
pupa (figure 160) hangs under twigs, so that its belly is above. The shading is brought about so that it matches exactly: the caterpillar gets lighter
from back to belly, the pupa from belly to back.

White animals find it especially difficult to hide their shadow (figure
154). Coloration alone cannot work, because for these animals a darker
coloring of the back would make them visible as dark spots in snow or
against the sky, and making the belly brighter than white is technically
impossible. But even here there are solutions. The heron in figure 162
is hung with long feathers on both sides of the neck and body, so that
at least the most conspicuous shadowy spots on the neck and belly are
occluded and, in addition, the revealing contour of the body is broken
up by the fringe of feathers.

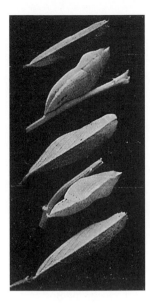

Figure 160

Two pupae of the clouded yellow butterfly (*Colias edusa*), laid for experimental purposes between alfalfa leaves. The upper one is wrongly illuminated from the back, the lower one correctly illuminated from the belly: above one sees a plump animal body, below an object like a bent leaflet (about natural size).

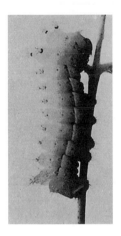 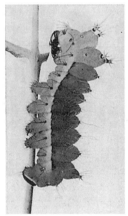

Figure 161

The caterpillar of *Actias selene* (a distant relative of the emperor moth). (a) With illumination from the back, roundedness is exaggerated: the animal almost seems to burst. (b) With illumination from the belly, its shape becomes completely disembodied.

The shading of the body, as suggested, achieves its purpose only under the right illumination; that is, for certain particular orientations of the body, namely, when the darkest part of the body—which in the higher animals is usually the back—is turned toward the light. Otherwise the volumetric effect of overhead illumination is only enhanced by the shading rather than canceled (figures 161 and 162, 163 and 164). This is also why live fish that swirl and tumble about in the water often look not merely dark, but often like disembodied shadows, similar to the

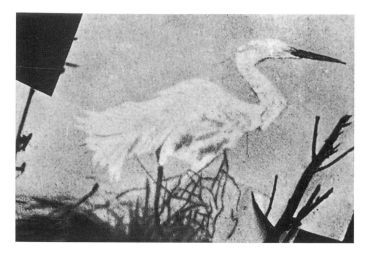

Figure 162

In white animals the belly shadow is often covered with overhanging feathers or fur hanging down on both sides. Model of a heron in mating plumage, photographed against the sky. (Figures 162–164 from Thayer; see figure 153.)

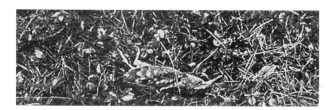

Figure 163

Woodcock, the same kind as in figure 71 (*Philohela minor*) lying dead on its back. The shading due to illumination and due to coloration now has the same direction, and the animal emerges perceptually as volumetrically rotund from its environment.

caterpillar in figure 161. But sick and dead fish that drift near the surface belly-up are not only radiantly bright, they appear doubly rounded and volumetric. Also in the garden when one is picking off caterpillars by raising and turning over twigs and leaves, not only are hidden animals thus exposed and ones that are sitting quietly startled, but the camouflage of animals sitting out in the open is unwittingly destroyed because they are rotated from the orientation in which their shading matches exactly the direction of illumination. For the same reason shading is useless for living creatures that constantly change their orientation. Apes that tumble

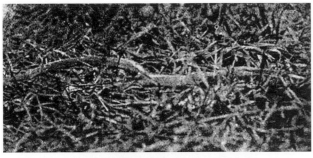

a

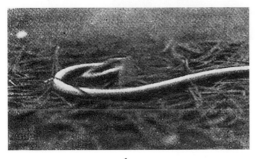

b

Figure 164
The snake *Liopeltis vernalis* (a) correctly on its belly is shadowy, and barely visible. (b) Lying on its back it is strikingly bright and volumetric. Explanation the same as in figures 160, 161, and 162.

about in the trees, and bears that often walk upright (not to mention humans) do not have countershaded hides.

4. ADAPTIVE BEHAVIOR

The reasoning developed above would suggest that animals that do use countershading would have to be constantly aware of how they should orient themselves so that their coloring does not have the opposite effect and deliver them into their enemies' fangs instead of concealing them. And indeed countershaded animals do behave as if they knew this. They are so disposed that they appear to be uncomfortable as long as their orientation does not match that for which shading becomes countershading and thus breaks up their shape most thoroughly.

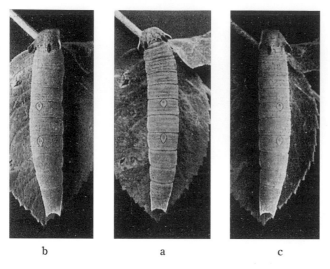

b   a   c

Figure 165
Caterpillar of the two-tailed pasha butterfly (*Charaxes jasius*) that is adapted (a) to illumination from the back, (b) when lit from the left inclines itself to the left, and (c)
correspondingly to the right. (Figures 165–170 from Süffert; see figure 159.)

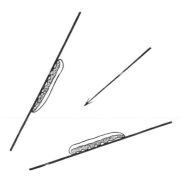

Figure 166
One caterpillar of the clouded yellow butterfly
(*Colias edusa*) hangs under the twig, the other
lies on top of it; both are oriented so that they
receive light (indicated by the arrow) from the
back.

For example, if you illuminate caterpillars of a great variety of species from various directions, they are observed universally to rotate to
bring themselves into the most advantageous orientation; that is, to position themselves with their darkest part turned toward the light and
their brightest part turned away from it (figures 165 and 166). This is
not always so simple (figure 167). When presented with a sudden change
of illumination some species of caterpillars (e.g., figure 161) twitch as if
they had been touched. In these caterpillars the sense of light is actually
much closer to the sense of touch than in the human; their photosensors

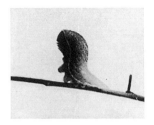

Figure 167
Caterpillar of the scarce swallow-tailed butterfly (*Papilio podalirius*) stands steeply erect, so that at least the anterior part of its body is oriented correctly to light coming in from the right.

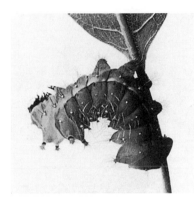

Figure 168
Suddenly the illumination comes from behind. The *Actias* caterpillar bends back as far as it can so that at least the lower side of its anterior end is turned toward the light. It would of course be better to crawl to the other side of the leaf stem, and indeed that is what the caterpillar does if illumination persists long enough from the new direction.

are not confined to the eyes, but distributed over the entire surface of the body. And the correct orientation with respect to illumination in these animals seems to depend primarily on these photosensors on the skin. Their behavior is not always the most appropriate in the first instant that the illumination direction is changed (figure 168), but that is no different in humans either. Even when caterpillars are illuminated from quite unnatural directions using special apparatus (figure 169), for example, from below, they quickly take on the orientation that is optimal for their camouflage (figure 170). They then appear to feel most comfortable in postures that no caterpillar of their species has ever held for extended periods. Such a fine interplay between the color of the body and the corresponding behavior could hardly have evolved without thereby conferring a particularly effective visual protection against all sorts of predators. As the animal experiment shows, the effectiveness of the now standard practice in camouflage of using irregular blotches of color could be amplified by carefully selected countershading not only of larger structures, but with objects of every size (cannon barrels, airplane fuselages, gasoline tanks, etc.) that are normally disposed in a

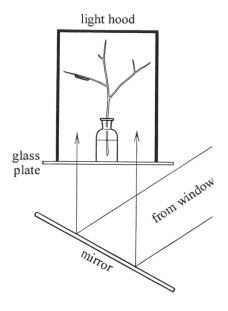

light hood

glass
plate

from window

mirror

Figure 169
Experimental set-up of Süffert to illuminate the caterpillars from below. Arrows represent light rays. The light hood (thick line) screens off all light that comes from above and from the sides.

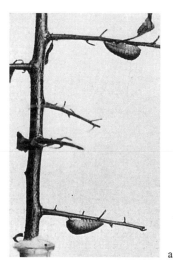
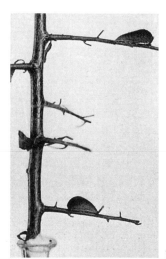

a   b

Figure 170
Two caterpillars of the scarce swallow-tailed butterfly (*Papilio podalirius*) that, as can be inferred from the dark coloring of its back, customarily sit on top of horizontal twigs of blackthorn. They were illuminated from below for a while, and therefore now hang from the underside of the twigs. (a) Now the illumination is changed to overhead lighting, and the caterpillars again look invitingly rounded, but not for long. (b) Half an hour later they are back on top of the twigs, and look flat like leaves.

horizontal orientation. Occasionally one finds on such objects a kind of countershading as a more or less accidental by-product of camouflage of a different kind. Perhaps one example is when an airplane fuselage is painted with dark earth colors to conceal it from view from above, and with the light colors of the sky to protect it from being seen from below. Systematic experiments in this direction would certainly be worthwhile.

11

The Wandering Moon

1. The Wandering Moon

When the moon becomes visible through moving clouds (figure 171), you often cannot avoid the impression that it is drifting in a direction opposite to that of the clouds; often the clouds even seem to stand still and only the moon is moving. One can make this observation not only on the moon or on the sun. The same effect occurs if you hold the point of a long pencil stationary over a sheet of paper that you slide back and forth (figure 172), or if you hold a fingertip against your forehead, with eyes closed, while turning your forehead back and forth. It also occurs that your whole self is dragged into this kind of illusory motion. When you look at a flowing current from a pier, the moving stream sometimes unexpectedly turns into a placid lake, and the pier becomes a moving vessel that seems to carry you off on a fast journey. This effect is most vivid when the sense of up and down is violated, as in the fairground ride known as the "Haunted Swing" [Translators' note: In German *Hexenschaukel*, literally "witches' swing"], in which the apparently ever wilder swinging bench-swing appears finally to swing all the way over the top, whereas in reality it is the entire structure of the surrounding room that swings and flips upside-down, while the bench-swing never moves from the spot (figure 173). This phenomenon is known as *induced motion*.

2. The Most Obvious Explanation

How does this illusion come about? The answer seems to be easy. In our experience it has always been swings that swing, and fortunately not houses; we let the pencil wander across the paper, not the paper under the pencil; and we certainly drew our hand across our forehead more often than our forehead over our hand. It might even seem like exaggerated thoroughness to continue to conduct specific experiments on this question. But if one does so, if one observes, for example, in a

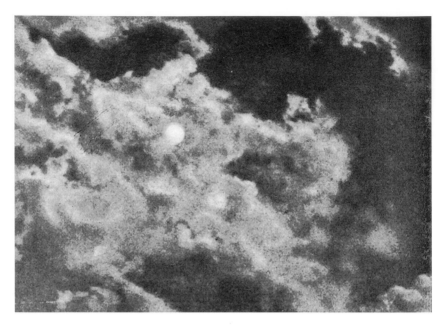

Figure 171
Do the clouds move past the moon or the moon past the clouds? Often it looks very vividly as though only the moon is moving. (Photo: Drei-Kegel-Verlag, Berlin.)

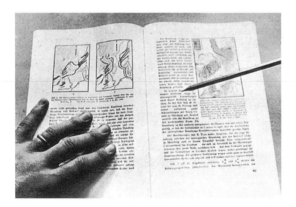

Figure 172
If you slide the paper back and forth, the pencil point seems to move.

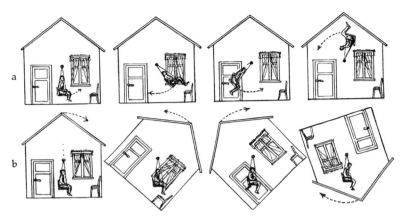

Figure 173
The haunted swing: (a) apparent, (b) actual movement. The house swings about the same axis as the bench-swing that it surrounds, and eventually flips all the way in a somersault. But the people sitting on the swing do not realize this, they feel as if they are swinging and turning upside down while the house is stationary, even though the bench-swing is the only thing that remains stationary.

completely dark room the picture of a house and a car, one of which is moved very slowly, then it is the car that seems to move, again consistent with our past experience, even when in reality it is the picture of the house that is moving (figures 174 and 175).[79]

3. MORE DIFFICULT CASES

But how does the explanation fit for the other cases, for example, for the sun and moon? It actually fits better than one might at first dare to hope. During our most impressionable age, in the first few years of life, the sun and moon catch our attention, for they always seem magically to move along with us as we walk, while everything else appears to fall behind.

The explanation is simple. The moon's distance from us is so enormous relative to the distances we cover while walking that the direction in which we see it remains completely unchanged in contrast to the visual direction of objects in our immediate environment (figure 176).

79. In such experiments nothing whatever but the two objects in question must be visible; even a barely perceptible glimmer of light can ruin the effect. The movement must always be very slow. Furthermore, for the best results, it is safer that the object that is expected to be seen in motion be kept stationary in reality. These conditions apply as well for all the later experiments discussed here.

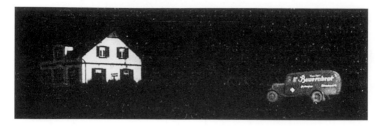

Figure 174
Experiment for testing the role of experience in a dark room. Two images are projected in a dark room from two projectors. Each can be moved independently. For example, in the experiment the image of the house is moved very slowly to the right. The observer does not notice this motion, but sees instead the truck moving to the left. (Figures 174, 175, 177, 181–184 from Walter Krolik: *Über Erfahrungswirkungen beim Bewegungssehen. Psychol. Forschg.* 20, 1934.)

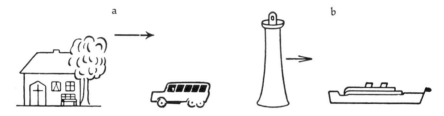

Figure 175
Even if you use quite primitive cartoon drawings instead of natural photos, you see (in the pure experiment) the vehicle moving, which is consistent with past experience, whereas in fact it is the building that is moving. (a) The house is moved to the right (arrow), while the vehicle appears to move to the left. (b) The lighthouse is displaced to the right and the ship seems to travel to the left. With slow movement in both instances the buildings seem to stand quite still. The surround in this and all following experiments is to be considered completely dark, as in figure 174.

But when you are sitting in a train at a railroad station, and think that your own train is moving when it is actually the neighboring train, past experience speaks neither for nor against this interpretation. And when a bridge on which you are standing appears to start moving relative to the flowing current, past experience would be expected to oppose this interpretation, except for the special case of a sailor or some other "water rat" who has gazed into the water hundreds of times from a moving ship. There must therefore be other explanations besides experience alone, and thus we cannot dispense with experiments after all.

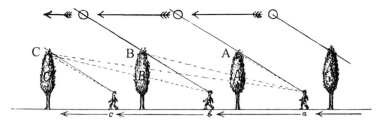

Figure 176
The visual elevation of the moon remains always the same as a result of its enormous distance. Thus the wanderer at point *a* sees it over tree *A*, at point *b* over tree *B*, etc. Wherever he goes, the moon always goes along with him.

Initially, these experiments should be performed using so-called experience-free stimuli—that is, stimuli for which the observer should have no bias due to experience, such as dots, lines, rectangles, and so on. For example, if you want to test whether the smaller of two different-sized objects tends to appear in motion—as might be assumed based on past experience—you might present the observer in the dark room with a large rectangle moving relative to a small dot of light (figure 177a). The result of this experiment is surprising, for usually it is the image at which the observer is looking that is perceived as the one that is moving. So in this case it is not the properties of the stimuli that are decisive, but rather the behavior of the observer.

This now raises a strong suspicion. Do we really know where we have been fixating in the examples involving past experience? Is it not most likely that our gaze was directed at the point at which we expected something special to occur, which would have been the vehicle? If so, then even in those cases past experience would not be the cause of the movement, but merely our choice of viewing direction. But this suspicion can be resolved. In the first place new experiments can be devised that draw the observer's gaze, as well as attention, to the building. For example, a continuously blinking light can be installed in the window of the house (figure 175a) and in the dome of the lighthouse (figure 175b), and while the observer is completely absorbed in this captivating event, the displacement begins unexpectedly. As a rule the observer nevertheless sees the *vehicle* move, just as before. So past experience is apparently a stronger factor than direction of gaze. Second, experiments with vehicles can be devised in which the direction of apparent motion is independent of the direction of fixation (figure 178). The image of the

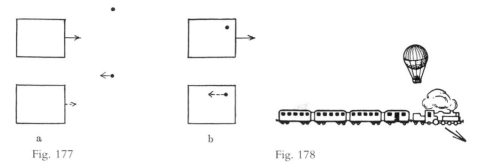

a   b

Fig. 177   Fig. 178

Figure 177
Movement experiment (in the dark) with experience-free objects. On top the actual movement: the dot is static and the rectangle is moving (arrow). At the bottom the apparent motion: (a) when the dot and the rectangle are adjacent to each other, the impression of movement alternates between the two figures. (b) When the dot is inside the rectangle, almost without exception it is perceived to move. Thus it is not size, but enclosedness that matters. (From Karl Duncker: *Über induzierte Bewegung. Psychol. Forschg.* 12, 1929.)

Figure 178
Experiment to test the effect of experience with exclusively mobile objects. The train is moved down toward the right (arrow), but it is perceived to move horizontally to the right. The vertical component of the movement is taken over by the balloon, which appears to rise vertically upward.

train is moved diagonally downward. According to past experience, trains travel only straight ahead, and the vertical component of the motion would then have to be adopted by the balloon. In fact, one either sees the train moving to the right while the balloon rises up vertically, or the train appears stationary, and only the balloon seems to move, obliquely upward to the left, both consistent with past experience.

4.   NEW DOUBTS AND THEIR RESOLUTION

Even in cases in which experience plays no role, there are circumstances in which the direction of fixation has no effect. If the rectangle (figure 177b) drifts across the dot, the dot alone appears to move as long as it remains inside the rectangle, even when you fixate on the rectangle as intently as possible. Even your own eyes now seem to remain fixed in one direction, while in reality they follow the movement of the rectangle; and conversely, they seem clearly to move as long as they are fixated on the dot (which really is stationary). Thus enclosedness may apparently

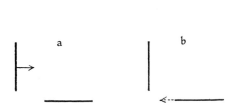

Figure 179
One does not generally include lines in the class of vehicles; nevertheless it happens that in a pure experiment one tends to move more readily, whereas the other more readily stands still. Here, for example, the vertical line is moved to the right (arrow) (a), but instead one sees the horizontal line, which extends in the direction of the movement, wander to the left (b).

accomplish what we expected earlier from size: in ambiguous cases the enclosing object tends to appear stationary, the enclosed object appears to be moving. When an object such as a pier, which is known to be firmly anchored, suddenly seems to start moving when nothing but rushing water is to be seen all around, that is the best proof that enclosedness is stronger than past experience. Another influence is seen from the *shape* of the objects, as shown in figure 179, where motion is perceived preferentially *parallel* to a line segment as opposed to *orthogonal* to it. Here it is again a matter of a law of organization, a Gestalt law that itself cannot be reduced to past experience any more than the other Gestalt laws can. Surely without this law, experiences with the moon and with the pencil, and especially with the haunted swing, would not be as impressive and insuppressible as they are.

But what about the experience in the train, where you think that your own train is starting to move, whereas in fact it is the neighboring train that is departing? Here everything you see through the window is after all undoubtedly framed by the window and the wall of your compartment (figure 180). By the law of *enclosedness*, if everything is not deceptive, the opposite should occur. When your own train is moving, it should seem as if the neighboring train is moving. And neither should we expect, by the same principle, that when viewing a movie of a scene photographed aboard a ship in a heavy sea, that suddenly instead of a heaving horizon on the screen, the whole auditorium seems to rock up and down. This occurs even when you sit in the last row and the screen occupies only a small part of your visual field. But does the window frame really enclose the landscape? In the retinal image it certainly does; but of course that is not the way we perceive it, it is only one of the causes of our perception. When we actually look out of the train window, the

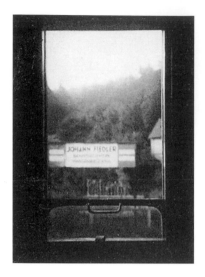

Figure 180
View from the train.

window frame certainly determines the section of the landscape that we see; but when it is not too small, we have a vivid sense that the whole of our train is only a small object embedded in the much larger landscape.[80] According to the law of enclosure, therefore, the train must appear to be moving, even when in reality the fortuitously visible part of the environment (the neighboring train) is in motion. But if you sit farther from the window and succeed in seeing the view as a kind of picture on the wall, the more the movement must be attributed to the landscape, until in the limiting case the landscape alone appears to be moving, and the train that is actually moving appears stationary. The experience in the cinema can be understood in the same way. For spectators who are at first so fully involved in the action that they no longer see a picture of the sea on the screen, the theater, no matter how large it might be, becomes small in contrast to the vastness of the sea, and must therefore begin to come into movement by the law of enclosedness. The self-motion must stop as soon as the spectators extricate themselves from the spell of the action and find their way back to reality.

Aside from the effect of enclosedness, there is a whole range of other immediate effects of the stimulus arrangement. Thus, long straight lines appear to move especially easily in their own direction (figure 179).[81]

---

80. This is one of the most impressive examples of the effectiveness of the perception of invisible entities [amodal perception]; See p. 135 section 8.

81. Compare p. 120, figure 129.

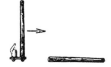

Fig. 181   Fig. 182

Figure 181
The short vehicle is not seen to drift downward any more than the long train in figure 178. So the result of the experiment in figure 178 was not due to the length of
the train, as one might have suspected from the experiment in figure 179.

Figure 182
Experience-free lines of the experiment shown in figure 179 are transformed into
familiar objects known from past experience. Now the one that is extended in the
direction of movement is usually no longer seen to move; rather, it is the one with
wheels that is perceived to move. Past experience is stronger than linear extension.

In contrast to physical theory of motion, in perception there thus
remains (1) a fundamental difference between rest and motion, and (2)
that motion is not at all relative; nor is it left up to the pleasure of the
observer. Rather it is determined by objective laws (more or less compelling depending on the circumstances) according to what is resting
and what is under way.

Now we return to experiments like those in figures 175b and 178
full of gloomy misgivings. Because besides past experience, it could just
as well have been the elongated Gestalt and its orientation that prompted
specifically the ship to appear moving and prevented the train from drifting downward [in figure 178]. The stock of past experience is falling
again. But all is not yet lost. Instead of the train we use a vehicle (figure
181) and watch to see whether or not a downward drift is now perceived
on it. In fact, the vehicle also appears to move only forward, not downward; and it is so short that one can no longer claim that its shape is the
cause. Encouraged by this success, we look for a new group of familiar
objects, arranged spatially and moved like the lighthouse and the ship,
but with the vertical object moving consistent with past experience
(figure 182). The vertical stimulus is a small electric cart with a tall tree
trunk standing vertically on it. And look, now it appears in most, but

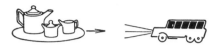

Figure 183
Limits of the effect of past experience I.
Surprisingly, in a straight experiment the
tea tray is perceived to move as easily
and as often as the vehicle (see text).

not all observations that the cart moves horizontally with its load. The
effect of past experience is thus again confirmed; here its influence is
somewhat stronger than that of spatial arrangement.

5.   POINT OF APPLICATION AND MODE OF ACTION OF PAST EXPERIENCE

Where does past experience act in motion experiments? One might be
inclined to wager: of course on the object with which we have past experience. We are acquainted with vehicles as being in motion, experiences of movement "cling" to them (are associated with them) and
because of this in ambiguous cases it is the vehicles that we tend to see
moving, whereas the experience of immobility clings to buildings with
corresponding consequences. But after so many surprises we have become accustomed to testing once again that which appears self-evident,
just to be on the safe side (figure 183). From the foregoing discussion it
follows compellingly that a vehicle should move and a tea tray should
remain stationary so long as no one picks it up. But once again our pre-
diction is wrong. For in this experiment it is sometimes the vehicle,
sometimes the tea tray, and sometimes both of them that are perceived
to move. If we had not already independently established the effectiveness of past experience, we might once again doubt its influence. So we
are left with the conclusion that the perception of motion does not cling
to individual objects, but to their *relationship with respect to each other*.

If we now look again—naturally not on the paper, but in the
darkened laboratory room—at our assemblies of familiar objects, what
we have vaguely suspected all along becomes clear. There is not just a
house and next to it a vehicle, but rather a vehicle in the midst of a
landscape in which by chance only the house is visible. The house is
not a single isolated item, but rather it represents to some extent the entire landscape through which the vehicle travels. The lighthouse does the
same thing, but naturally not the tea tray.

Now we can also surmise how past experience really works here.
First, there are not two past experiences at play, one that moves the vehicle and one that holds the house still. And second, past experience is

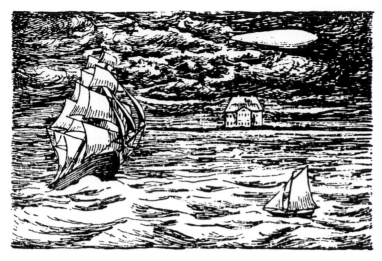

Figure 184
Limits of the effect of past experience II. Mobile objects (clouds, waves, ships, airship) are the ones that are actually in motion here; but in the direct experiment it is the house that is perceived to be in motion (see text).

not at all concerned with moving and holding still. Experience contributes only the invisible landscape to the house, and that landscape includes the vehicle. *Everything else then is done by the law of enclosedness*, according to which the landscape lies fixed, along with the house, and the vehicle moves within it. Even an invisible environment, as we know, can very well have such definite effects.

Now once again a test with an experiment. The surround of a house is filled so thoroughly with moving things—water, clouds, airship, sailboats (figure 184)—that no space remains for completion by past experience. The stretch of coastline on which the house stands is so narrow that it hardly carries any weight. For this experiment the observer must be placed so close to the picture that most of the visual field is filled with the moving objects. Now past experience is shown to be ineffective. The environment seems to stand still, but the house, the only object that should not be able to do this, glides about in clear and lively fashion as if this were the most natural thing in the world.

6. CONCLUSION

Past experience has been established as an independently active force, at least for the motion phenomena that have been investigated. But this result did not come quickly and effortlessly, as was assumed in the last two centuries, when for every striking phenomenon one came up immediately with theories of past experience and considered further testing in such cases unnecessary. Furthermore, we must be clear that we can no longer view past experience as the single all-encompassing basis for explanation even in other areas of perception. Its role then has become more modest; it can now be counted as one among various other sometimes very powerful forces that have their origin partly in Gestalt relationships and partly also in the condition and behavior of the observer.

The enormous significance of the constantly growing stock of earlier experiences in the life of humans and of higher animals can hardly be overlooked. Perception itself is also improved through use, practice, and schooling[82] and makes possible an increasingly finer, richer, and deeper grasp of things. But these facts should not be permitted to blind us to the idea that the fundamental laws of perception are present before the accumulation of this stock of experience, and before such schooling. Those fundamental laws are not profoundly changed by experience, but rather, without the existence and stability of these laws, the store of past experience could neither be collected nor utilized. The generally held view that everything in perception except for the raw sensory qualia of colors, tones, and the like is derived first and foremost from past experience, is based in turn not on expert knowledge, but rather on assertions that were fabricated at their desks by philosophers of the so-called age of enlightenment, and this view turns out immediately to be untenable under closer scrutiny. The heat and passion with which past experience theories in our field are being defended is, aside from the question of what is fact, hard to comprehend. For to be based on past experience, or more correctly, based on habit, after all means nothing other than imposed externally by force. Is the thought that with regard to the most essential things our senses should conform to laws that are externally imposed on them really that much more worthy of a human being, and so much more attractive than the possibility, at least equally likely and obvious, that they operate according to laws that have their origin in our own nature?

---

82. It should be mentioned in passing that active, volitional practice and experience in perception are completely different from the habit that is driven mindlessly by perpetual repetition, as suggested by theories of experience.

12

Laws of Seeing and Laws of Nature

1. The Laws of Seeing as Mental Laws

Are the laws of seeing *psychological* or *physiological* laws? We have not as yet posed this question. But has it not been answered indirectly? If during the course of the investigation the so-called judgment theory of perception were proven false and inapplicable[83] and the influence of attention and of past experience or habits were shown to be so limited that it would be impossible to base a general theory of perception on them without some kind of conjuring tricks,[84] is anything else left but a physiological explanation? Our answer to this question is that we can indeed think of something quite different; for why should the possibilities of the mental be exhausted with the functions of judgment, attention, and habit? That is a prejudice of textbook psychology from which we must free ourselves.

The organization of the visual field occurs within us essentially without our involvement, and without our explicit awareness of any of its laws. But when we come to understand these laws through our research on the visual processes, we feel at ease: in a realm of meaningful events, in the realm of the intellect and not in the realm of lifeless machines, blind chance, and senseless coercion, suggested by associationist theories that explain everything by habit and experience. We feel, if we had been at liberty to create the order in the visual field (under prevailing stimulus conditions) for ourselves, we could scarcely have done it better or more sensibly.

---

83. Especially chapters 6 and 7.

84. On attention theory compare esp. chapter 2, pp. 15, 27; chapter 4, p. 43. On theory of experience, chapter 2, p. 15; chapter 3, p. 29; chapter 9, p. 145; and primarily all of chapter 11.

2.   RELATED LAWS IN OTHER MENTAL DOMAINS

Not only generally, but even in specific details, we find similar laws and principles active in domains of experience and behavior where there is no question that these are mental domains. We see this in imagination and cognition.

When a military commander makes global sense of a confused battlefield situation based on dozens of individual reports and observations, or a judge forms a picture of a crime from a confusion of eye-witness reports and questionable evidence, when from such various reports, those that fit together into a self-consistent story are rendered prominent, while those that appear insignificant and have no relevance to the case are rejected, clearly it is the law of *greatest order* that is at work (chapters 2 and 3). Just as with the grouping percepts in figure 36 or the laws of camouflage in chapter 5, this law can also lead to compelling and yet false conclusions in the cognitive realm; for example, in an apparently airtight, but nonetheless faulty case of circumstantial evidence. With a change of viewpoint in thinking we often find the same unstable alternations between conclusions as seen in figure 54, and the addition of new evidence can promote the same irrevocable kind of reorganizations as seen in figure 34. And we have every reason to consider these processes as fundamental to productive thinking.[85]

The law of greatest order manifests itself just as much in cognition as it does in vision. When among the confused jumble of fragments of conversation at the dinner table those that belong together seem to find each other, while the extraneous ones seem to drop out, this occurs by the same laws (and is prevented probably for the same reasons) as the perceptual separation of colored surfaces in the case of transparency (chapter 8, figure 131), as can be demonstrated experimentally. When we later recall all of the various overheard conversations neatly sorted and segmented in our memory, this is clearly related to the perceptual segmentation of closed, differently constructed parts of figures as observed in peripheral vision (chapter 8, figure 144). Furthermore, when a historian while examining an old manuscript, or a geologist while inspecting rock strata, gets the impression that there must be a gap and infers exactly what seems to be missing and how it would have to continue, the relationship to the laws of overlapping (chapter 8, fig-

---

85. Compare W. Köhler: *Intelligenzprüfungen an Menschenaffen*, 2nd ed. Berlin, 1921, and Wertheimer: *Schlußprozesse im produktiven Denken*. Berlin, 1920.

ure 138) in vision is clear. Finally, when in the memory of long-ago experiences, in rumors, and legends passed on through oral tradition, inappropriate portions are gradually deleted and distorted, doubtful portions are straightened out and made to fit together, gaps are filled, characters simplified and unified, and more clearly segregated from each other, and in general, that which is striking and essential is emphasized ever more strongly, and occasionally exaggerated beyond measure, then we remember that improvements of the same kind occur on a smaller scale unintentionally wherever observations are made under unfavorable conditions (chapter 8, figures 142–145).

The connection between perceptual Gestalten under unfavorable observation conditions (with loosely articulated stimuli) and true memories can be seen in afterimages and even more clearly in eidetic images that appear to play a major role in the lives of some people, especially in the prepubescent years, as discovered and investigated by E. R. Jaensch. With these phenomena it is possible to observe the real object initially under favorable conditions and then to remove it. The initially strong and clearly distinct stimulus disappears suddenly and completely, but without the visual image also disappearing immediately and permanently, as is the case in normal adults. With some observers who are capable of eidetic imagery, quite remarkable changes are observed in these persistent images as they morph toward greater regularity and uniformity of the character, which they can track directly (unlike changes in memories and Gestalt deviations that result from loosely articulated stimuli that almost always are already in their final regular shape). The fact that these changes are not seen by normal observers despite favorable conditions is probably less due to Gestalt forces being weaker in those people, than to the material on which these forces operate being more resistant.

Among the first words of a small child was the expression *abbutz* which meant *schmutzig* ["dirty"]—*abputzen!* ["wipe off"] and *beschädigt (kaputt)* ["broken"]—*heil machen* ["fix it!"] all in one. The underlying meaning of order and unity of substance and form could not be more impressively demonstrated than through the early occurrence of this comprehensive term. When children, while playing with blocks and stones, are initially occupied exclusively with sorting similar items together and are perhaps annoyed if the resulting groups do not come out to equal size, and when playing with boxes of buttons and nails, carefully sort out everything that is made of a different material, or is a slightly different shape, you can immediately recognize the transition from laws of perception to laws of behavior. It has sometimes been said that in the study of the Gestalt, psychology has slipped into a foreign domain: it is concerned not with laws of perception, but rather, with laws of artistic creation. That might be going too far: in 11 chapters we dealt only with plain seeing, seeing of objects and events as we find them when we just open our eyes. But there is doubtless a deep connection between the natural striving of the senses for greatest order and unity, and the human urge to produce order and unity among things in the environment far beyond the order that is absolutely necessary, and to create new forms of greatest inner harmony and compactness of structure.

Let us just briefly point to another domain of mental life in which not only humans participate: the grouping, linking together of living beings themselves. "Birds of a feather flock together," even the wording is reminiscent of the law of similarity. If the relationship to that law of seeing is more than a passing resemblance, we should expect from the outset that it is only one of many laws of grouping of living creatures. In fact it is not just the black hen that is expelled from a flock of white hens, but also the fifth wheel [in a social group] feels clearly uncoupled. Finally, who is not reminded of our figure 47, when one sees how differences among people that can lead to sharp disputes lose their divisive influence as soon as these people encounter a stranger?

3.   THE UNIVERSAL APPLICABILITY OF THE LAWS OF PERCEPTION

Of course, many readers might have missed what is often considered an unavoidable sign of psychological laws: the emphasis of typological, that is, genetically based, differences, and the establishment of a system of the various inherited types of seeing.

We have not forgotten nor do we mean to underestimate these differences. We saw above how, for example, in the creation of perceptual units in countless stimulus distributions a competition emerges among a number of good alternative groupings, each with its own virtues, but the relative weights of these different organizations are not always the same across individuals (chapter 4, figures 59–63). But it was not possible to understand these individual differences correctly until the general law was found that constitutes their common basis. This applies to the theory of perception in general as well as to psychology overall.

A psychologist can focus on describing different types of individuals, to bring them into a system and devise procedures by which they are rapidly and correctly identified. Practical considerations at this point in history make this branch of psychology especially urgent. But this is, as we said, only one branch of psychology. As in the biological sciences, besides the description of different species, besides zoology and botany, experimental biology has been added as a necessary independent science to investigate that which is common among living organisms in general. So too typological psychology requires an experimental psychology that concentrates entirely on the investigation of common general laws of the psyche as a necessary complement.

Furthermore, there is today no lack of practical reasons for concentrating on the commonalties of mental life. How would it be possible to achieve even a scanty understanding of the most external and everyday things, let alone a common enterprise, to enable the creation of societies with a unified direction of will, if mental life was not based on a very broad and secure basis of common responses to the environment? It would be a task for a poet to portray the confusion that would result if this common basis of perception in a group of people were suddenly to disappear, leaving only the differences between individuals that are described in typology doctrines.[86]

4.   LAWS OF SEEING IN HIGHER ANIMALS

A recent study of animal camouflage concludes with the comment: "This is how animal camouflage affects us as human beings; whether it works the same way for animal predators, we do not know." In the meantime careful experiments have shown that animals with protective camouflage in the appropriate environment escape their animal predators (birds) just as they do from us humans (cf. figure 95a), and in an inappropriate environment are just as much more easily detected by them as by us. The Gestalt laws on which camouflage depends must therefore also apply for these birds.

In experiments with various species of birds, for example jays, the validity of individual Gestalt laws has been directly demonstrated, specifically the laws of similarity (of color and size), of proximity, and of good continuation (figure 185). Higher animals (apes, chickens, parrots), like humans, manifest the phenomena of brightness and color constancy

---

86. Compare chapter 2, esp. figure 16f.

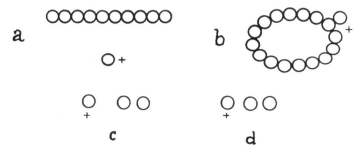

Figure 185

Test of laws of organization in the jay. The circles represent small overturned pots; while the bird is watching, something edible is hidden under one of them for the bird to retrieve later. (a) Many identical pots, one of them placed farther away from the others. When food is hidden under this one, it is never missed (law of proximity or segregation through distance). (b) Pots placed next to each other without any space between them in a ring, with one pot outside the ring. If food is hidden under the surplus pot it is immediately recognized, but not so for the pots in the ring (segregation of the item that does not fit in with good continuation). From M. Hertz: *Wahrnehmungspsychologische Untersuchungen am Eichelhäher. Z. vgl. Physiol.* 7, 1928). (c) and (d) Testing the limits of the effectiveness of distance differences: in (c) the single pot standing alone is still reliably approached, but no longer in (d).

under varying illumination (chapter 6), of size constancy with changing distance, and of shape constancy with varying location (chapter 7).

With chickens it was possible to demonstrate the phenomena of color contrast and even the existence of various optical illusions (figure 186). Rats and mice recognized shapes across variations in material substance: when they had learned that a black triangle on a white ground was the sign for food, they recognized it again, as we do, when it was a white triangle on a black ground, or when it was drawn only in outline, and even when the triangular outline had gaps (figure 187).

Dogs and even fish (minnows and sticklebacks) see a movie essentially as we do: they see movement where in reality a rapid sequence of still pictures is presented. Only with the completely different eye structure of the fly does this effect no longer occur.

In contrast, the movement law of enclosedness (chapter 11) seems to be valid even with flies. As with the person in a haunted swing, flies behave as if they were being rotated in space, when in reality it is only the walls surrounding the space in which they are positioned that are being rotated (figure 188). Even here it appears to be a matter of a particularly deep-seated conformity to law.

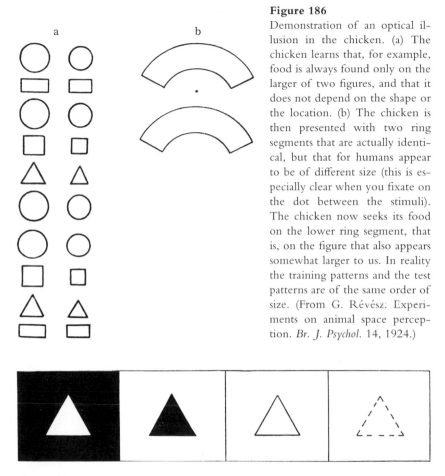

Figure 186
Demonstration of an optical illusion in the chicken. (a) The chicken learns that, for example, food is always found only on the larger of two figures, and that it does not depend on the shape or the location. (b) The chicken is then presented with two ring segments that are actually identical, but that for humans appear to be of different size (this is especially clear when you fixate on the dot between the stimuli). The chicken now seeks its food on the lower ring segment, that is, on the figure that also appears somewhat larger to us. In reality the training patterns and the test patterns are of the same order of size. (From G. Révész: Experiments on animal space perception. *Br. J. Psychol.* 14, 1924.)

Figure 187
Images that even a rat recognizes as similar. (From K. S. Lashley: Basic neural mechanisms in behavior. *Psychol. Rev.* 37, 1930.)

Despite fundamental commonalties, naturally the world will look very different for different animals. For a bird, for example, that feeds on grain, tiny dotlike objects will play a much more important role in the organization of their visual field than for a human or a large beast of prey. If a bird finds its nourishment in dark crevices, the boundary effect whereby small differences in color are suppressed by neighboring stronger differences may not be as influential as it is in humans. We pointed out further important differences in chapter 4. But none of this changes the universal commonalties of the basic laws.

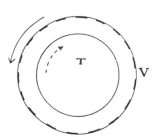

Figure 188
Test of the laws of motion perception in animals. The inner circle T is (seen from above) a table on which, for example, a fly sits under a glass bell jar; the outer circle V is a curtain with vertical black and white stripes. If only the curtain rotates (outer arrow), the fly behaves as if the table were being turned in the opposite direction (dashed arrow). So even for the fly it seems that the motion law of enclosedness (chapter 11) applies. (From M. Gaffron: *Untersuchungen über das Bewegungssehen bei Libellenlarven, Fliegen und Fischen. Z. vgl. Physiol.* 20, 1934.)

5. INADEQUATE PHYSIOLOGICAL EXPLANATIONS

If certain basic laws of seeing apply this far down into the animal kingdom, we are again faced with the question whether these are not natural laws after all, that is physiological laws; in other words, laws that can be found not only from within, from experience, but basically also from outside, through investigation of sensory organs and the nervous system.

It is already established that what textbook psychology calls physiological explanations are as worthless as its so-called psychological explanations. Neither from the structure of the eyes and the inherent relationships of refraction and their resulting image formation, nor from the structure of the retina with its resolution as based on an enormous number of pointlike stimulus receptors, nor from the fibrous structure of the higher brain areas would one ever have come to the formulation of the laws that we have demonstrated above in our visual experiences. On the contrary, knowledge of physiology has again and again obstructed and diverted the discovery and recognition of the actual laws of seeing.

But how about explanations involving the properties and habits of eye movements? There is hardly any prominent property of shape perception and perceptual segmentation that someone has not yet tried to attribute to eye motions; this was proposed most recently, for instance, for the law of good continuation. For some time it was even believed that we really do not see the basic shapes of things at all, but become aware of them only by eye movements made while exploring those shapes visually.

Here naturally the first question arises: do you really sense your own eye movements clearly and precisely enough for this? As we already found in chapter 11 (p. 150), that is not the case. To convince yourself, you should stand in front of a mirror, look into the eyes of your mirror image, and turn your head side to side. Not only do you see your head movements, you also feel them very clearly. Of the eye movements themselves you feel virtually nothing, even though you see clearly that they are just as extensive as the head motions.

Ocular behavior indicates a similar conclusion. If you try to trace a circle, a rectangle, and an S with your eyes, your eyes move in paths that are not even close to similar to the intended pattern (figure 189), even if you have the feeling that you have traced it correctly. When the same person tries to do this repeatedly, the errors do not become any smaller. From this it follows that if we depended on evidence from our eye movements, in figure 189 we would not be able to distinguish the curves within each column, nor between them, and the target figures above them. This means we would confuse the shape of a circle with that of a potato or a withered leaf!

The decisive clue came through an experiment of nature.[87] A man became mentally blind [visual agnosia] after an occipital head injury in the war. He could no longer immediately recognize visual forms; however, he was still able (as before) to feel most precisely his own voluntary eye movements. This man was still capable of following visual lines with movements of his head (although not of his eyes) and thereby recognize the shape of the lines by the shape of these movements, exactly as predicted for normal perception according to the eye movement theory of shape perception.[88] In this way the agnosic patient could even read written text, as long as nobody held his head to prevent it from moving. But besides the fact that his performance was very slow, he experienced peculiar difficulties that are entirely foreign to the normally sighted. If he started to trace a letter at the wrong end, he could not recognize it (figure 190). If you crossed out a word that he had just read

---

87. Compare p. 3.

88. It speaks in support of the essential relationship between the laws of seeing and those of natural thinking (2nd section of this chapter) that this mentally blind man could no longer think perceptually like a healthy person. For example, he was no longer capable of understanding metaphorical expressions, but nevertheless could reach logical conclusions by the familiar processes of reasoning learned in school. In mathematical calculations he could produce the result only by counting, as taught in the fundamentals of arithmetic that specify calculation sequences (addition, subtraction, multiplication, and division). Cf. W. Benary: *Studien zur Untersuchung der Intelligenz in einem Fall von Seelenblindheit. Psychol. Forschg.* 2, 1922.

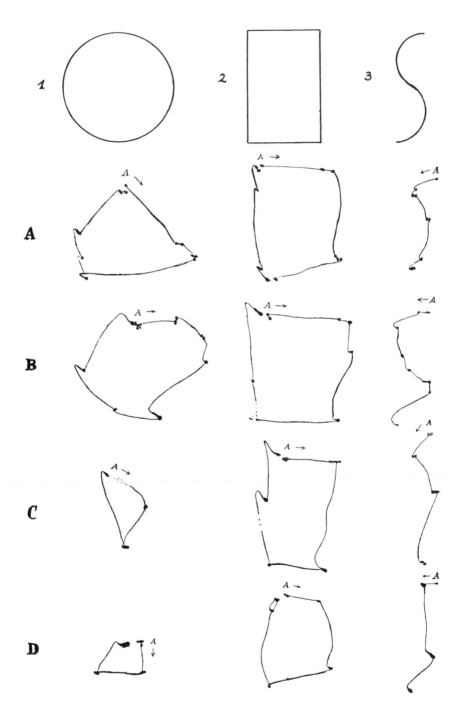

successfully, using a line of the same ink as the script, he could no longer decipher it. He continuously went astray and thereby produced a confused movement trace of totally unknown form derived partially from the word and partially from portions of the crossing line (figure 191).

This means that you cannot follow a shape at all with eye movements if it is not segregated beforehand from its surround by other factors. Such other factors must be present in normals[89]; otherwise they would necessarily have the same problems in seeing visual form as the mentally blind person.

It should be noted: If head or eye movements that are actually performed cannot lead to reliable shape recognition, it is completely implausible that mere shifts of attention[90] and other virtual movements that are only intended but never actually carried out could do any better. Theories that appear, even today, in some psychological writings are strongly reminiscent of the story of the little girl standing next to her mother and audibly murmuring the Lord's Prayer. "You already know the Lord's Prayer?" asks the mother after church. "Oh yes!" says the girl. "Then say it for me again!" "I can't do it. I can only do it silently."

6. ON THE QUESTION OF THE POSSIBILITY OF ALSO DERIVING THE LAWS OF VISION PHYSIOLOGICALLY

Processes that come closest to true vision take place far from the eyes in the cerebral cortex. We will have to understand the nature of this domain if we want to have any prospect of approaching the laws of vision from the outside by the physiological route.

---

89. Compare also the recognition of shapes by touch, chapter 4, figure 66.

90. Healthy persons moreover almost never perform this without corresponding eye and head movements, if they do not happen to be performing perceptual psychological experiments.

◀ **Figure 189**
Photographic records of eye movements during tracing of curves with the eyes. On top are test patterns, below them are eye movement curves; the two lowest rows are from an experiment in which the observer attempted to retrace the curves from memory with the eyes on an empty blackboard. Our impression that we are able to follow such curves with our eyes exactly and with smooth motion is absolutely deceptive, as revealed by these traces. (From G. M. Stratton: Eye movements and the aesthetics of visual form. *Philos. Studien.* 20, 1902.)

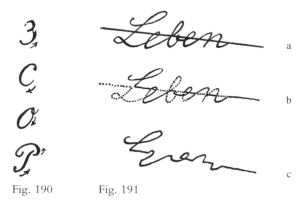

Fig. 190   Fig. 191

Figure 190

When the mentally blind person [visual agnosic], who can recognize only the shape of his own head movements, traces a letter in the wrong direction, he does not recognize it. He says of the "C", it is an arc; with respect to the "3", this is two arcs attached to each other; with respect to the "O", a ring and a short line on it, etc. (Figures 190 and 191 after Gelb and Goldstein: *Psychologische Analysen hirnpathologischer Fälle I. Zur Psychologie der optischen Wahrnehmung und des Erkennungsvorgangs.* Leipzig, 1920.)

Figure 191

If someone such as the mentally blind person must trace the handwriting to recognize written words, he can no longer decipher a word that has been crossed out (a). For him the law of good continuation is no longer effective, he is consequently constantly in danger of going astray at intersections (b). The path of his eye movements therefore bears no resemblance to the crossed-out word (c). Hence the law of good continuation is not a law of eye movement.

That the brain consists of a tangle of fibers and cells is not, however, the most fundamental observation. That is also true in some sense of a telephone exchange, yet all comparisons of the cerebrum with a complicated switchboard have always led to error.

More fundamental is the fact that, like the entire living body, the cortex is a system of finely distributed fluids. Not switches and electrical wires, but air bubbles floating in a coffee cup, and drops of fat floating on soup (among many others) belong among the kind of structures whose behavior we must investigate in order to obtain information about the possibilities [neuronal correlates] of visual events in the brain. The science of these structures is, of course, scarcely older than psychology itself, and the expert would answer most of the questions a psychologist might pose with: "Quite possible, but we have not investigated that yet." But one thing is already abundantly clear. Of the known results of this science, so far none significantly contradicts the observations of perceptual theory. On the contrary, the similarity is often so striking that one can hardly consider it accidental. The examples that follow of course concern only some of the most crude and simple phenomena; and nothing would be more premature and more foolish than to believe that the mind–body problem would be solved through these examples.

The formation of a sharp border between two differently colored areas is reminiscent of the formation of a boundary surface between two fluids. Not every pair of dissimilar fluids develops a sharp boundary where they meet; water and oil do so, but not water and alcohol. Similarly, not every pair of dissimilar colors develops a sharp border; sometimes even the largest contrast in hue [equiluminant colors] generates nothing but a blurry transition stripe, unless the two colors also differ in brightness (figure 192).

In every boundary surface (not just between fluids) a surface tension force exists that seeks to shrink that surface. It is the force to which soap bubbles owe their spherical form. The strength of that force increases as the size of the bubble is reduced. In microscopically small bubbles surface tension finally overpowers all other shaping forces. That is why even crystals below a certain very small size always have rounded-off corners, and still smaller ones are round like a droplet. A very similar phenomenon is observed when visible objects become sufficiently small: their shape becomes ever more rounded. Finally they become rounded dots, often long before their image becomes as small as a retinal cone, and when they are not sufficiently enclosed they decompose into groups of little dots (figure 193).

Even the formation of bridging lines (chapter 3), and the filling in of gaps between small adjacent structures in the visual field can be reproduced in a fluid model (figure 194). Furthermore, we can only hint suggestively at the similarity between the contrast of figure and ground in vision (chapter 1) and the contrast between closed phase (drops of fat) and open phase (soup) in fluid systems. Just as in perception, in fluids the closed phase has especially strong pattern forming forces: the shape of the drops of fat is strictly rounded, although their location, by which the shape of their environment is after all determined, is virtually arbitrary (aside from the effect of specific gravity).[91]

---

91. Strictly speaking the latter is valid only for drops floating freely in the interior of another fluid, not for those that are suspended from the boundary surface of two other fluids (water and air).

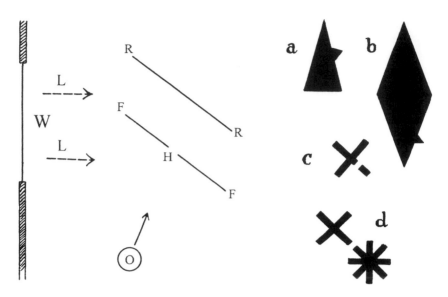

Figure 192

Setup for blurring of border lines between two colors of the same brightness [equiluminant colors]. W is the window with incoming light (L = direction of incident light). To the right of it, the diagonal lines represent two sheets of colored paper, for example, the one green, the other red; the front one (F-F), with a cut-out figure (H) in the middle, is fixed, the rear one (R-R) is held by an assistant and slowly rotated to vary the brightness of the reflected light, until the edges of the hole fade for observer (O) (at a sufficient distance). The hole must be carefully cut out with a sharp knife on a firm surface, so that no light or shadow lines arise on its edges. Because of the visibility of the cut edges, cardboard is not suitable for this experiment. The most effective shapes are pointed. With shapes like (a) and (b) the extra parts disappear most easily; the meaningless gap in the cross (c) disappears much more easily than the equally large interspace between cross and star (d). Both correspond with the results described in chapter 8. (From S. Liebmann: *Über das Verhalten farbiger Formen bei Helligkeitsgleichheit von Figur und Grund. Psychol. Forschg.* 9, 1927.)

With this we have come to our last examples: to the striking beauty and regularity of the shape of fluid membranes in equilibrium, which are especially reminiscent of the regularities of the depth effect of perspective drawings (chapter 7), and to the way that fluids seek their own level in a fixed container (chapter 8).[92]

We must be clear that in these examples it is only for now a matter of agreements of a very general kind, and that in no case has it been shown whether a real relationship exists as opposed to just an accidental

92. Compare Köhler: *Die physischen Gestalten.* Braunschweig, 1920.

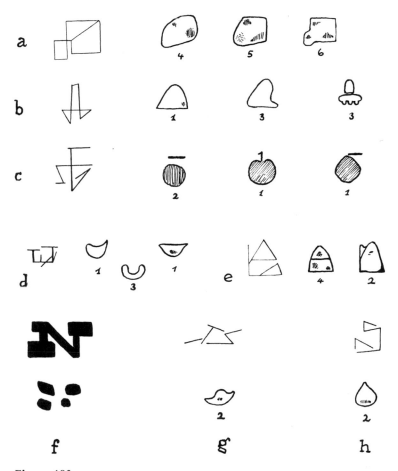

Figure 193

Rounding-off of the very smallest perceivable objects. The test figures (with the exception of the N), the observation conditions, and the significance of the numbers are the same as in figure 142. The rounding-off occurs for some observers more easily and with larger figures than for others. In (c) and (f), besides rounding, the figures are observed to break up into several individual blobs. (The N is from C. Berger: *Zum Problem der Sehschärfe*. Dissertation, Berlin, 1932. Everything else is from E. Wohlfahrt, copied; see figure 142).

Figure 194

The Pleiades. Fluid model for the bridging over gaps in the perception of compact dot figures. Sodium hydrate drops on hydrochloric acid gelatin, with litmus as indicator. (From R. E. Liesegang: *Cassinotaxis, Eine scheinbare Fernwirkung bei Diffusionen.* In: Dessauer: *Zehn Jahre Forschung auf dem physikalisch-medizinischen Grenzgebiet.* Leipzig, 1931.)

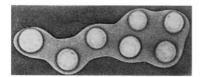

similarity. But that does not diminish the value of these suggestive analogies, nor does it exempt us from the task of further investigation [of continuous, analog, fieldlike processes in the brain]. We should do this with redoubled confidence, given that for the main basis of experience theory, the so-called association-by-contiguity, which a short time ago was viewed fairly generally as a certain matter of fact, no analog has been found so far in all of nature. We know of no natural law according to which two arbitrary materials, objects, or events, if they are only brought into contact often, long, and strongly enough, finally adhere to each other for any prolonged period of time. On the contrary, this result is achieved only in nature, as in perception, always entirely by characteristics of the two structures in their mutual relationship.[93] With the right characteristics you do not even need to bring the structures into contact, they strive by themselves to approach each other and often come together across considerable distances.

7.   AN APPARENT CONTRADICTION AND ITS RESOLUTION

Can we really do justice to the laws of seeing? Will we not do violence to them, and let the best and most important of them fall by the wayside, if we try to advance toward these laws by the physiological route? This sort of thinking has happened often enough in psychology; you only have to think of the still widely held view that visual objects are permitted to have only those properties that, according to our knowledge of image formation in the eye, are already possessed by the retinal image. But this danger would exist only if we restricted ourselves exclusively to psychological phenomena that we can infer from our presently

---

93. Compare Köhler: *Psychologische Probleme.* Berlin, 1933; chapters 4 and 8, esp. p. 177.

incomplete knowledge of the physical and chemical interactions in the nervous system, based on physical and chemical laws that by chance happen to have already been established.

Have we done this anywhere? On the contrary: we have proceeded exclusively and without a side glance into physics, chemistry, anatomy, and physiology, from within, from the immediate percept, and without even thinking of rejecting any aspect of our findings or even just changing its place, just because it does not fit with our contemporary knowledge of nature so far. With our perceptual theory we do not bow to physiology, but rather we present challenges to it. Whether physiology will be able to address these challenges, whether on its course, by external observation of the body and its organs, it will be able to penetrate to the laws of perception, is pointless to argue about in advance.

But is this dispute, without our noticing it, not already decided? Have we not ourselves emphasized in the first place that we view the laws of seeing as well as certain laws of imagination, thinking, creating, and behavior throughout as mental laws? And did we not contradict our own assumptions most grossly when we soon thereafter turned to consider whether these mental laws might not indeed also be physiological laws, that is, natural laws? Our answer is no. Both approaches, mental and physical, are equally important for us.

The mental and physical laws come into conflict only if we cling to the opinion that the human spirit is a stranger in this all-too-petty physical world, and also a stranger in the physical body that sadly must for some time be our prison, and to whose laws we only submit with reluctance. But this opinion is neither self-evident nor proven, but simply, for almost a millennium and a half, has been handed down and believed within the framework of traditional theological doctrine. To this day it has had a profound influence on philosophical and scientific thinking, even where (as in enlightenment philosophy) one presumed oneself to be independent of this doctrine, or even to contradict it.

This has been the tacit presupposition of all "past experience theories" of perception. For if you assume that the spirit itself emerged directly out of nature with which it must cope, it is quite conceivable, indeed it is even most reasonable, to assume from the outset that mind conforms to the essential properties of nature fittingly and meaningfully, and thus mind and brain need not first accommodate to each and every property of physical nature. It is also at the heart of Kant's subjectivism, namely, of the opinion that the character and law of human experience cannot for this reason be the character and law of ultimate reality. It is also the cause of the old-fashioned horror that seizes some philosophers when they hear the claim that it should be possible to build a bridge between our knowledge of the mental and our knowledge of nature.

It is just as valid, however, to adopt the opposite presupposition— that even our spirit, and with it our perceptual experience, is an integral part of nature. True, it is a very special and certainly not the simplest part of nature, but in any case it is the only one that is immediately given to us. Every other science must satisfy itself with indirect copies and representations of things, and those representations emerge in us only at the end of a long and complicated chain, by way of light waves or sound waves, through stimulus receptors on the body's surface, and through longer or shorter neural pathways, along which a good deal of information is lost along the way, or filtered out or distorted through the processing laws of the transmitting media. If this is so, then surely psychology offers more reliable information about the essence of being than any other realm of knowledge, if we only try to look at things correctly and do not let ourselves be led astray by the limited and indirect information of other sciences.

The conviction that this is how the matter stands is the deepest reason why we study psychology and perceptual science.

Index